DEDICATION

To all my beautiful readers

Disclaimer

The information in this book is not to be used as medical advice and is not meant to treat or diagnose medical problems. The information presented should be used in combination with guidance from your physician.

TABLE OF CONTENT

OUTSMART CANCER

Introduction

There is simply no denial to the universal fact that health comes from holistic "natural" living. This holistic approach includes but is not limited to healthy expressions of feelings, complete harmony with the nature, love and care from the surroundings (inner and outer), and above all wholesome nutrition and hygiene. In summary, we can say living as close to the Mother Nature as possible while keeping away from the various artificial toxins is the key to a healthy and long life.

Latest research reveals that almost 85% of all the cancer cases are somehow related to the following three major groups of risk factors:

- Unhealthy Nutrition - this includes a high cholesterol, high sugar, a high fat and low fiber diet.
- Unhealthy Lifestyle - this includes unhealthy habits such as smoking, drinking alcohol, depression, stress and sedentary lifestyle.
- Unhealthy Environment - this includes chemical carcinogens, industrial toxins, air and water pollution, electromagnetic radiations.

Health, even when compromised by cancer due to any of the above mentioned risk factors, can be restored and healing can be achieved by re-establishing the holistic approach to cancer treatment. There are countless cancer-victors who have defeated cancer by harmonizing and balancing their body, mind, spirit and emotions.

It is important for you to note that cancer can be defeated by using natural compounds and modalities in conjunction with the conventional therapy or as a standalone therapy. This e-book will guide you through the logic behind this approach and how to use natural diet as an effective tool against cancer. It will guide you through the safest and most effective cancer treatment alternatives known today. You will be able to learn how to use various herbs, shrubs, vegetables, fruits, and supplements, plus specialized new substances such as **Vitamin B17** (commonly known as Amygdalin or Laetrile), shark cartilage, and many other to prevent and reverse cancer. This is probably the most helpful book for those who actually want to live a cancer-free life.

Chapter 1

FOOD FOR THOUGHT

When it comes to treating cancer one statement fits in perfectly "prevention is better than cure". The very fact, that there are no proven reasons behind the occurrence of cancer makes us all vulnerable to this deadly disease. It can strike anyone at anytime, whether you are prepared for it or not. Prevention of cancer is therefore of prime importance and needs to be addressed to make sure you do not get it in the first place. In order to better prepare yourself to fight effectively against cancer; you need to make sure you need everything about cancer. Because the more you know about the various aspects of this deadly disease, the more informed and educated decisions you will be able to make about cancer treatment and cancer prevention.

Some interesting facts about Cancer

If you think you know everything about cancer, you need to think again. Following are some of the interesting facts about cancer most of us do not have any idea about.

1. The chances of survival rates (cure rates) for the same kind of cancer vary greatly depending on the kind of treatment option selected and range from 3% to 90%. The harsh reality is that most of us use (are pushed to use) the 3% cure rate treatment option because most of are unaware of the 90% cure rate cancer treatment options.

2. The cancer treatment options that offer 90% cure rate have the potential to revert cancer cells into normal cells.

3. The cancer treatment options that offer 90% cure rate are inexpensive, safe and gentle and have existed for decades. The irony is that only a limited number of people know anything about these treatments.

The next obvious question that strikes in our minds is that why such helpful information is not available to the cancer patients and why they are pushed to use the cancer treatment options that offer only 3% cure rates?

If you are unable to come out with right answer to the above questions, let me open your eyes to another harsh reality of life, the **Patents**. All of us are programmed in such a way that we are forced to use only the "Patented" drugs/products for treating our cancer. There are many stakeholders behind this Patent business who make huge profits by selling the drugs. For them money is more important than the survival of the cancer patients, therefore they do not let the other cancer treatment options come to the lime light that offer the 90% cure rates.

This eBook is intended to provide you access to the cancer treatment options which offer **90% cure rates** and are never discussed in any electronic or print media channels. The reason for the low publicity of such alternative cancer treatments is that the people who endorse such treatment options have limited budget to influence the media or the Congress or anyone in the higher circles. The only information you get about such treatment options is through some websites and some publications/research work.

This eBook is designed in such a way that you will not feel the urge to go visit any other website or go to any library to find everything about the various alternative ways for treating or preventing cancer. Instead of focusing on the traditional ways to cancer treatment, this eBook focuses on the holistic approach of cancer treatment and cancer prevention.

Once you are done reading this comprehensive eBook on Caner Prevention and Cancer Treatment using all natural ways, you will be in a better position to make a decision whether to go for the traditional approach of cancer treatment of combine it with the alternative options to get maximum benefits and increase your chances of survival.

Before going into further details about topic of Cancer Prevention and Cancer Treatment, it is mandatory to shed some light on various aspects of this fearsome disease that claims the lives of hundreds of thousands of people across the globe every year.

Chapter 2

CANCER – WHAT YOU NEED TO KNOW

Cancer continues to be one of the leading causes of death even in the most medically advanced and highly industrialized countries of the world, despite the fact that billions of dollars are spend each year on the research, diagnosis and treatment of this deadly disease. It is estimated that one out of three persons will die of some sort of cancer in the coming years.

How well do you know about the #2 killer disease in the world is a million dollar question, despite the fact that tons of information is available both online and offline on the topic. While reading the following lines, keep in mind that there are many different forms of cancer and every case is unique, so you will never be able to learn each and everything about Caner in just a few lines. However, you will surely learn a lot more in respect to working knowledge about cancer. Questions like:

- Who is at risk?
- What factors contribute in increasing the chances of cancer at large?
- What can you do to stay cancer-free?

Although most of the facts about cancer treatment and cancer prevention are common sense, but the fact of the matter is "common sense in not so common". Knowing so much about cancer and knowing that certain lifestyle choices can increase your risk of developing cancer; most of us do not act until it is too late.

Let us have a look at some of the cancer facts that everyone should and must keep in mind to increase the odds of living a cancer-free life.

- Did you know that one out of every eight person dies of cancer in the world every day? An astonishing finding is that developed countries have a higher rate of such deaths, and the cause is linked to a combination of diet and lifestyle.

- Once referred to as a "wasting disease", cancer actually represents more than 100 diseases. Cancer develops as a result of the abnormal growth and multiplication of the some body cells, which damage healthy cells of the body along the way. Except the cancer that affects the blood, most types of cancer result in tumors.

- There is a general consensus among the cancer researchers worldwide that at least half of the cancer related deaths are preventable. As per their calculations, as much as 1.6 million deaths will occur in 2015 due to cancer, and saving half of them i.e. 0.8 million can make a great difference and give people some hope that they can lead a normal life once again.

- Latest research also shows that only a small proportion (about 5% or less) of cancer can be linked to genetics. Next time you hear some say your cancer is genetically linked; you have the latest statistics to prove it otherwise.

- Environmental factors play an important role in increasing your risk of getting cancer. The food you eat, the air you breathe and the water you drink, all play an important role in exposing you to getting cancer. Most of us spend a big chunk of our time at home, office or schools, so ensuring proper hygiene and personal safety should be give top most priority.

- Most of us link tobacco to cancer; however this is not actually the case. It is believed that 90% of all the lung cancer is caused by smoking. Latest research reveals that it is not tobacco that causes the cancer; rather it is the chemicals that are used in the process of making tobacco products. Lung cancer is the leading cause of death among men and women living in the world, it is estimated that one person dies from lung cancer every thirty seconds. Even the second hand smokers are at great risk of developing lung cancer.
- Did you know that sleep deprivation can also be a source of developing cancer? Well, according to the latest research, insomnia or lack of sleep can increase your chances of developing colon cancer. Research conducted on the people who work night shifts shows that they are at a higher risk of developing colon cancer. Well, next time you think about sleeping, make sure to enjoy at least 8 hours of un-interrupted sleep.
- Another surprising fact for you; more than 4 children will die of cancer today. Cancer is the number one killer of children. The irony is that children cannot be exposed to the conventional cancer treatment methods, such as Chemotherapy and radiation therapy, as both of these methods are actually cancer causing.
- Did you ever try to read the label of the hot dogs or sausages or any other processed meat packet? I beat you did not, well next time you should. Most of the processed meat items contain nitrates in the form of sodium nitrate or potassium nitrite, which work as preservatives and also add flavor. When confronted with heat and the digestive fluids presented in the stomach, these nitrates are converted into nitrite, which is a carcinogen.

- Another every day product that we use without any caution is the sunscreen. Most of the people believe that exposure to sun increases your chances of developing cancer; however this is not completely true. Exposure to sunlight is actually beneficial to the skin as the sunrays help the body to produce vitamin D, which is good for healthy skin and strong bones. The actual cause of developing cancer is your sunscreen. Most of the sunscreens actually work against you, as they disperse the beneficial UV light and cause the skin to burn - leading to the development of cancer. In addition to that most of the sunscreens also contain a chemical compound labeled as OMC (octyl methoxycinnamate) which becomes a toxin when it interacts with the sunlight. Some other chemicals such as dioxybenzone and oxybenzone are also extremely hazardous for your body as once they are absorbed in to the blood stream the generate free radicals, a potential cause of systemic cancer.
- Women are more prone to developing breast cancer and it is the leading cause of death among them.
- Men are more prone to developing lung, colon and prostate cancer and it is the leading cause of death among men.
- People of older age are more prone to cancer. As much as 75% of all the cancer patients are 55 or older.
- Obesity is also linked to increasing your chances of getting cancer.
- It is very hard to diagnose cancer in the early stages of development, therefore yearly screening is imperative, if you want to be on the safe side.
- Last but not the least, all the energy, resource and time is wasted in finding an effective treatment of cancer rather than finding the root cause of the disease. the

- Good news in the end, there are certain types of foods that have the ability to target and destroy the cancer cells. Food items such as kale, turmeric, berries, avocados, green tea, garlic and even dark chocolate have a tendency to reverse your cancer.

Stay tuned to learn something more interesting about the best alternative cancer treatments cancer patients are using effectively to cure and prevent cancer.

Alcohol

The general consensus scientifically is that alcohol is the lesser of two evils when compared to tobacco. However it has proven links to various types of cancer including cancers of the oral cavity (excluding the lips), pharynx (throat), larynx (voice box), esophagus, liver, breast, colon, and rectum.

And quite simply, the more you drink the higher the risk.

In an ideal world it's best to simply avoid alcohol however for most people the solution tends to be reduction and drinking in moderation infrequently.

As there is a direct link between the amount a person drinks to their risk of cancer, anything that can be done in the area of reducing alcohol consumption is welcomed.

So that leaves us with the primary topic of this book – you're food intake, essentially what is responsible for a poor diet or being overweight.

Exercise

While 40% of Americans will eventually develop cancer, only 14% of active Americans will get cancer. A half hour of exercise every other day cuts the risk for breast cancer by 75%. Exercise imparts many benefits, including oxygenation of the tissues to thwart the anaerobic needs of cancer cells. Exercise also helps to stabilize blood glucose levels, which can restrict the amount of fuel available for cancer cells to grow. Exercise improves immune function, lymph flow, and detoxification systems. Exercise helps us better tolerate stressful situations. For cancer patients who are able to participate, exercise improves tolerance to chemotherapy. Some therapists use hydrogen peroxide or ozone to oxygenate the tissue. Humans evolved as active creatures. Inactivity is an abnormal, under-oxygenated metabolic state--so is cancer.

Distress

It was the Canadian physician and researcher, Hans Selye, MD, who coined the term "the stress of life", so he could document the physiological changes that took place in lab animals when exposed to noise, bright lights, confinement, and electric shocks. The thymus gland is a pivotal organ in immune system protection against infections and cancer. Dr. Selye noted that stress induces thymus gland shrinkage, increases fats in the blood (for the beginnings of heart disease), and erodes the stomach lining (ulcers).

Since the 1920s, scientific evidence has been advancing the theory that emotional stress can depress the immune system and make that individual more vulnerable to infections and cancer. It was Norman Cousins' book, ANATOMY OF AN ILLNESS, that thrust this mind-body principle in front of the public. After 10 years of lecturing and researching at the University of California at Los Angeles, Cousins' theories held valid under scientific scrutiny.

Carl Simonton, MD, a radiation oncologist, found that his mental imagery techniques seemed to produce better results with fewer side effects for his cancer patients. In a study published in the British Medical Journal, scientists found that women who had experienced a "severe" stressful life event had a 1,500% increase in the risk of developing breast cancer. Bernie Siegel, MD, a Yale surgeon, found that certain mental characteristics helped his cancer patients to recover. Candace Pert, PhD, a celebrated researcher at the National Institutes of Health, discovered endorphins in human brains and led the charge toward unravelling the chemical mysteries of the mind. Dr. Pert says that the mind is a pharmacy and is continuously producing potent substances that either improve or worsen health. Since the mind can create cancer, it should seem a logical leap that the mind can help to prevent and even subdue cancer. Noted physician and researcher at the University of California San Francisco, Kenneth Pelletier, MD, PhD, wrote his groundbreaking book, MIND AS HEALER, MIND AS SLAYER, to show that certain personalities are more prone to certain diseases. Many alternative therapists use a wide variety of psychological approaches to help rid the body of cancer.

Clearly, there is some mental link in the development of cancer for many patients. I have worked with many cancer patients whose major hurdle was spiritual healing. While dietary changes are difficult for many people, it is far easier to change the diet or take some nutrient pills than change the way we think. Pulling emotional splinters is a painful but essential experience. Not only is there a metaphysical link to cancer, but the site of the cancer may provide clues regarding how to fix the problem. Many breast cancer patients have experienced a recent divorce, which results in the loss of a feminine organ. One patient of mine suffered from cancer of the larynx, which began one year after his wife left him with the thought "there's nothing you can say that will make me stay." If spiritual wounds started the cancer, then spiritual healing is an essential element for a cure.

Toxic overload

Of the 5 million registered chemicals in the world, mankind comes in contact with 70,000, of which at least 20,000 are known carcinogens, or cancer-causing agents. Each year, America alone sprays 1.2 billion pounds of pesticides on our food crops, dumps 90 billion pounds of toxic waste in our 55,000 toxic waste sites, feeds 9 million pounds of antibiotics to our farm animals to help them gain weight faster, and generally bombards the landscape with questionable amounts of electromagnetic radiation.

Bruce Ames, PhD, of the University of California at Berkeley, has estimated that each of the 60 trillion cells in your body undergoes from 1,000 to 10,000 DNA "hits" or potentially cancer-causing breaks every day. Newer studies examining the role of the immune system in protecting us against cancer show that the average adult has one cancer cell appear each day. Yet somehow, for most of us, our DNA repair mechanisms and immune system surveillance are able to keep this storm of genetic damage under control. Wallowing in our own high-tech waste products is a major cause of cancer in modern society, since carcinogens add to the fury of the continuous assault on the DNA. Noted authority Samuel Epstein, MD, of the University of Illinois, says that a major thrust of cancer prevention must be detoxifying our earth. Toxins not only cause DNA breakage, which can trigger cancer, but also subdue the immune system, which then allows cancer to become the "fox in the chicken coop", with no controlling force.

Early research indicated that once cancer has been upregulated, or "the lion is out of the cage", then no amount of detoxification is going to matter. Newer evidence says otherwise. Cancer growth can be both slowed and even reversed, under the right conditions. According to the National Cancer Institute, there are 7 million Americans alive today who have lived 5 or more years after their cancer diagnosis. Cancer is reversible. If toxins caused the problem, then detoxification is the solution. For more on detoxification, see the chapter on changing the underlying causes of cancer.

Chapter 3

THE CAM APPROACH FOR CANCER TREATMENTS – A GLIMPSE

Since most of you already know about the various conventional cancer treatment methods, which only interfere with cancer's ability to grow and spread, so there is no need to dig deep into such options, since they only offers 3% cure rates. This chapter is intended to provide you information about different other ways you can use to treat cancer in combination with or without undergoing radiation therapy, chemotherapy or any other form of conventional cancer treatment, this approach to cancer treatment is most commonly referred to as CAM approach or Complementary and Alternative methods used to treat/prevent cancer.

Most of the people intermix the two terms, complementary cancer therapy and alternative cancer treatment, whereas both of them are two different approaches. Complementary cancer therapy is used in conjunction with the conventional cancer treatment, where as alternative cancer treatment therapies are used in place of the conventional treatment options. This difference needs to be clear in your minds, before reading any further.

Complimentary Therapies

Following are some of the complementary therapies that are offered to the cancer patients undergoing conventional cancer treatments, to ease their pain and suffering from different symptoms and make them stronger physically, mentally and emotionally.

- Acupuncture
- Exercise
- Aromatherapy
- Hypnosis
- Massage Therapy
- Music Therapy
- Meditation
- Yoga

Patients are better able to cope physically and emotionally with cancer and its side effects and enjoy a normal and pain free life, once they undergo such complementary cancer therapies.

Alternative Therapies

When it comes to alternative cancer treatment options, it is a totally different ball game. These are the treatment options that remain ignored by most of us, intentionally or unintentionally, in favor of drugs, radiation and surgery. As opposed to the conventional cancer treatment options, the alternative treatments are:

- successful
- low cost
- non-toxic
- all-natural

People who are either afraid of or do not doubt the effectiveness of the conventional cancer treatment options look towards alternative therapies.

Some of the alternative cancer treatment options, which offer promising results, are as under:

- Laetrile (Vitamin B17)

16

Laetrile is also known as amygdalin or as Vitamin B17 is the cancer treatment world. It is a substance which is derived from various nuts or pips of many fruits. Apricot pips or kernels are considered to be a good source of this cancer fighting substance. You may also be able to find it plants such as sorghum, lima beans or clover.

- The Gerson Therapy

People also refer it as Gerson diet, Gerson method or Gerson regime. It is actually an alternative cancer therapy diet. The main purpose of taking this highly nutritious diet consisting of nutritional supplements is to rid the body of the toxin and strengthen the immune system naturally.

- Shark Cartilage

Yes, you heard it right; there are many cancer patients out there who have benefited from this alternative therapy. The shark cartilage is available in the form of power, which is produced by grinding the cartilage taken from a hammerhead shark or a spiny dogfish shark.

Why CAM?

After reading such interesting and helpful information about the CAM approach for cancer treatments, you may be wondering why people with cancer prefer this type of approach over the conventional methods. Well, let me share with your some of the solid reasons why people prefer the CAM approach:

✓ People have lost faith and hope in the conventional cancer treatment options
✓ People are scared to experience the various side effects offered by the conventional cancer treatment options

- ✓ People are scared to taking all those medications and pills
- ✓ People want to take an active role in improving their own health and wellness.
- ✓ People like to remain close to the nature; they want to treat their cancer with their own will power, mind, body and things found in the nature.
- ✓ Some find the CAM approach to be simple, wholesome and without any side effects.

One thing that needs to be kept in mind is that the various techniques and products used in the CAM approach have been studied extensively and have showed promising results to fight cancer and make you feel better during your cancer treatment.

IN the end it is you, who has to make the final call, whether to become part of the conventional treatment system or go with the nature to treat your cancer. This book is an effort to provide you with all the information that you may ever need to make a good final decision when the time comes.

Chapter 4

THE ULTIMATE TEST

A look at the many cultures around the world that are, or have been, free from cancer; and an analysis of their native foods.

The best way to prove or disprove the vitamin theory of cancer would be to take a large group of people numbering in the thousands and, over a period of many years, expose them to a consistent diet of rich nitriloside foods, and then check the results. This, surely, would be the ultimate test.

Fortunately, it already has been done.

In the remote recesses of the Himalaya Mountains, between West Pakistan, India, and China, there is a tiny kingdom called Hunza. These people are known world over for their amazing longevity and good health. It is not uncommon for Hunzakuts to live beyond a hundred years, and some even to a hundred and twenty or more. Visiting medical teams from the outside world have reported that they found no cancer in Hunza.

Although presently accepted science is unable to explain why these people should have been free of cancer, it is interesting to note that the traditional Hunza diet contains over two-hundred times more nitriloside than the average American diet. In fact, in that land where there was no such thing as money, a man's wealth was measured by the number of apricot trees he owned. And the most prized of all foods was considered to be the apricot seed.

One of the first medical teams to gain access to the remote kingdom of Hunza was headed by the world-renowned British surgeon and physician Dr. Robert McCarrison. Writing in the January 7, 1922, issue of the journal of The American Medical Association, Dr. McCarrison reported:

The Hunza has no known incidence of cancer. They have ... an abundant crop of apricots. These they dry in the sun and use very largely in their food.

Visitors to Hunza, when offered a fresh apricot or peach to eat, usually drop the hard pit to the ground when they are through. This brings looks of dismay and disbelief to the faces of their guides. To them, the seed inside is the delicacy of the fruit.

Dr. Allen E. Banik, an optometrist from Kearney, Nebraska, was one such visitor. In his book, Hunza Land, he describes what happened:

My first experience with Hunza apricots, fresh from the tree, came when my guide picked several, washed them in a mountain stream, and handed them to me. I ate the luscious fruit and casually tossed the seeds to the ground. After an incredulous glance at me, one of the older men stooped and picked up the seeds. He cracked them between two stones, and handed them to me. The guide said with a smile: "Eat them. It is the best part of the fruit."

My curiosity aroused, I asked, "What do you do with the seeds you do not eat?"

The guide informed me that many are stored, but most of them are ground very fine and then squeezed under pressure to produce a very rich oil. "This oil," my guide claimed, "looks much like olive oil. Sometimes we swallow a spoonful of it when we need it. On special days, we deep-fry our chappatis [bread] in it. On festival nights, our women use the oil to shine their hair. It makes a good rubbing compound for body bruises."

In 1973, Prince Mohammed Ameen Khan, son of the Mir of Hunza, told Charles Hillinger of the Los Angeles Times that the average life expectancy of his people is about eighty-five years. He added: "Many members of the Council of Elders who help my father govern the state have been over one hundred."

With a scientific distrust for both hearsay and the printed word, Dr. Ernst T. Krebs, Jr., met with Prince Khan for dinner where he queried him on the accuracy of the LA. Times report.

The prince happily confirmed it and then described how it was not uncommon to eat thirty to fifty apricot seeds as an after-lunch snack. These often account for as much as 75,000 International Units of vitamin A per day in addition to as much as 50 mg of vitamin B17. Despite all of this, or possibly because of it, the life expectancy in Hunza, the Prince affirmed, is about eighty-five years. This is in puzzling contrast to the United States where, at that time, life expectancy was about seventy-one years. Even now, more than two decades later, life expectancy at birth in the U.S. is only about seventy-six.

That number may sound pretty good, but remember that it includes millions of old people who are alive but not really living. The length of their lives may have been extended by surgery or medication, but the quality of their lives has been devastated in the process. They are the ones who stare blankly into space with impaired mental capacity, or who are dependent on life-support

21

mechanisms, or who are confined to bed requiring round-the-clock care. There are no such cases buried in the statistics from Hunza. Most of those people are healthy, vigorous, and vital right up to within a few days of the end. The quality of life is more important than the quantity. The Hunzakuts have both.

It will be noted that the Hunzakut intake of vitamin A may run seven-and-a-half times the maximum amount the FDA allows to be used in a tablet or capsule, while that agency has tried to outlaw entirely the eating of apricot seeds.

The women of Hunza are renowned for their strikingly smooth skin even into advanced age. Generally, their faces appear fifteen to twenty years younger than their counterparts in other areas of the world. They claim that their secret is merely the apricot oil which they apply to their skins almost daily.

In 1974 Senator Charles Percy, a member of the Senate Special Committee on Aging, visited Hunza. When he returned to the United States he wrote:

We began curiously to observe the life style of the Hunzakuts. Could their eating habits be a source of longevity? ...

Some Hunzakuts believe their long lives are due in part to the apricot. Eaten fresh in the summer, dried in the sun for the long winter, the apricot is a staple in Hunza, much as rice is in other parts of the world. Apricot seeds are ground fine and squeezed for their rich oil, used for both frying and lighting.

And so, the Hunzakuts use the apricot, its seed, and the oil from its seed for practically everything. They share with most western scientists an ignorance of the chemistry and physiology of the nitriloside content of this fruit, but they have learned empirically that their life is enhanced by its generous use.

Five or six excellent volumes similar to Dr. Banik's have been written by those who have risked their lives over the treacherous Himalaya Mountain passes to gain entrance to Hunza. Also, there have been scores of magazine and newspaper articles published over the years. They all present the identical picture of the average Hunza diet. In addition to the ever-present apricot, the Hunzakuts eat mainly grain and fresh vegetables. These include buckwheat, millet, alfalfa, peas, broad beans, turnips, lettuce, sprouting pulse or gram, and berries of various sorts. All of these, with the exception of lettuce and turnips, contain nitriloside or vitamin B17.

It is sad to note that, in recent years, a narrow road was finally carved through the mountains, and food supplies from the "modern world" have at last arrived in Hunza. So have the first few cases of cancer.

In 1927 Dr. McCarrison was appointed Director of Nutrition Research in India. Part of his work consisted of experiments on albino rats to see what effect the Hunza diet had on them compared to the diets of other countries. Over a thousand rats were involved in the experiment and carefully observed from birth to twenty-seven months, which corresponds to about fifty years of age in man. At this point the Hunza-fed rats were killed and autopsied. Here is what McCarrison reported:

During the past two and a quarter years there has been no case of illness in the "universe" of albino rats, no death from natural causes in the adult stock, and, but for a few accidental deaths, no infantile mortality. Both clinically and at post-mortem, examination of this stock has been shown to be remarkably free from disease. It may be that some of them have cryptic disease of one kind or another, but if so, I have failed to find either clinical or microscopic evidence of it.

By comparison, over two thousand rats fed on typical Indian and Pakistani diets soon developed eye ailments, ulcers, boils, bad teeth, crooked spines, loss of hair, anemia, skin disorders, heart, kidney and glandular weaknesses, and a wide variety of gastrointestinal disorders.

In follow-up experiments, McCarrison gave a group of rats the diet of the lower classes of England. It consisted of white bread, margarine, sweetened tea, boiled vegetables, canned meat, and inexpensive jams and jellies—a diet not too far removed from that of many Americans. Not only did the rats develop all kinds of chronic metabolic diseases, but they also became nervous wrecks. McCarrison wrote:

They were nervous and apt to bite their attendants; they lived unhappily together, and by the sixteenth day of the experiment they began to kill and eat the weaker ones amongst them.

It is not surprising, therefore, to learn that westernized man is victimized by the chronic metabolic disease of cancer while his counterpart in Hunza is not. And lest anyone suspect that this difference is due to hereditary factors, it is important to know that when the Hunzakuts leave their secluded land and adopt the menus of other countries, they soon succumb to the same diseases and infirmities—including cancer—as the rest of mankind.

The Eskimos are another people that have been observed by medical teams for many decades and found to be totally free of cancer. In Vilhjalmur Stefanson's book, Cancer: Disease of Civilization? An Anthropological and Historical Study, it is revealed that the traditional Eskimo diet is amazingly rich in nitrilosides that come from the residue of the meat of caribou and other grazing animals, and also from the salmon berry which grows abundantly in the Arctic areas. Another Eskimo delicacy is a green salad made out of the stomach contents of caribou and reindeer which are full of fresh tundra grasses. Among these grasses, Arrow grass (Triglochin Maritima) is very common. Studies made by the U.S. Department of Agriculture have shown that Arrow grass is probably richer in nitriloside content than any other grass.

What happens when the Eskimo abandons his traditional way of life and begins to rely on westernized foods? He becomes even more cancer-prone than the average American.

Dr. Otto Schaefer, M.D., who has studied the diets and health patterns of the Eskimos, reports that these people have under- gone a drastic change in their eating habits, caused indirectly by the construction of military and civilian airports across the Canadian Arctic in the mid-50's. These attracted the Eskimos to new jobs, new homes, new schools—and new menus. Just a little over one generation previously, their diet consisted almost entirely of game and fish, along with seasonal berries, roots, leafy greens and seaweed. Carbohydrates were almost completely lacking.

Suddenly all of that changed. Dr. Schaefer reports:

When the Eskimo gives up his nomadic life and moves into the settlement, he and his family undergo remarkable changes. His children grow faster and taller, and reach puberty sooner. Their teeth rot, his wife comes down with gallbladder disease and, likely as not, a member of his family will suffer one of the degenerative diseases for which the white man is well known.

There are many other peoples in the world that could be cited with the same characteristics. The Abkhazians deep in the Caucasus Mountains on the Northeast side of the Black Sea are a people with almost exactly the same record of health and longevity as the Hunzakuts. The parallels between the two are striking. First, Abkhazia is a hard, land which does not yield up a harvest easily. The inhabitants are accustomed to daily hard work throughout their lives. Consequently, their bodies and minds are strong right up until death, which comes swiftly with little or no preliminary illness. Like the Hunzakuts, the Abkhazians expect to live well beyond eighty years of age. Many are over a hundred. One of the oldest persons in the world was Mrs. Shirali Mislimov of Abkhazia who, in 1972, was estimated to be 165 years old.

The other common factor, of course, is the food, which, typically, is low in carbohydrates, high in vegetable proteins, and rich in minerals and vitamins, especially vitamin B17.

The Indians of North America, while they remained true to their native customs and foods, also were remarkably free from cancer. At one time, the American Medical Association urged the federal government to conduct a study in an effort to discover why there was so little cancer among the Hopi and Navajo Indians. The February 5, 1949, issue of the Journal of the AMA declared:

The Indian's diet seems to be low in quality and quantity and wanting in variety, and the doctors wondered if this had anything to do with the fact that only 36 cases of malignant cancer were found out of 30,000 admissions to the Ganado Arizona Mission Hospital. In the same population of white persons, the doctors said there would have been about 1,800.

Thirty-six cases compared to eighteen hundred represents only two percent of the expected number. Obviously, something is responsible.

Dr. Krebs, who has done exhaustive research on this subject, has written:

I have analyzed from historical and anthropological records the nitrilosidic content of the diets of these various North American tribes. The evidence should put to rest forever the notion of toxicity in nitrilosidic foods. Some of these tribes would ingest over 8,000 milligrams of vitamin B17 (nitriloside) a day. My data on the Modoc Indians are particularly complete.

A quick glance at the cancer-free native populations in tropical areas, such as South America and Africa, reveals a great abundance and variety of nitriloside-rich foods. In fact, over one-third of all plants native to these areas contain vitamin B17. One of the most common is cassava, sometimes described as "the bread of the tropic." But this is not the same as the sweet cassava preferred in the cities of western civilization. The native fruit is more bitter, but it is rich in nitriloside. The sweet cassava has much less of this vital substance, and even that is so processed as to eliminate practically all nitrile ions.

As far back as 1913, Dr. Albert Schweitzer, the world-famous medical missionary to Africa, had put his finger on the basic cause of cancer. He had not isolated the specific substance, but he was convinced from his observations that a difference in food was the key. In his preface to Alexander Berglas' Cancer: Cause and Cure (Paris: Pasteur Institute, 1957), he wrote:

On my arrival in Gabon in 1913, 1 was astonished to encounter no cases of cancer. I saw none among the natives two hundred miles from the coast.... I can not, of course, say positively that there was no cancer at all, but, like other frontier doctors, I can only say that, if any cases existed, they must have been quite rare. This absence of cancer seemed to be due to the difference in nutrition of the natives compared to the Europeans....

The missionary and medical journals have recorded many such cancer-free populations all over the world. Some are in tropic regions, some in the Arctic. Some are hunters who eat great quantities of meat, some are vegetarians who eat almost no meat at all. From all continents and all races, the one thing they have in common is that the degree to which they are free from cancer is in direct proportion to the amount of nitriloside or vitamin B17 found in their natural diet.

In answer to this, the skeptic may argue that these primitive groups are not exposed to the same cancer-producing elements that modern man is, and perhaps that is the reason they are immune. Let them breathe the same smog-filled air, smoke the same cigarettes, swallow the same chemicals added to their food or water, use the same soaps or deodorants, and then see how they fare.

This is a valid argument. But, fortunately, even that question now has been resolved by experience. In the highly populated and often air-polluted State of California there are over 100,000 people comprising a population that shows a cancer incidence of less than fifty per cent of that for the remaining population. This unique group has the same sex, age, socioeconomic, educational, occupational, ethnic and cultural profile as the remainder of the State's population that suffers twice as high an incidence of cancer. This is the Seventh Day Adventist population of the State.

There is only one material difference that sets this population apart from that of the rest of the State. This population is predominantly vegetarian. By increasing greatly the quantity of vegetables in their diet to compensate for the absence of meat they increase proportionately their dietary intake of vitamin B17 (nitriloside). Probably the reason that this population is not totally free from cancer—as are the Hunzakuts, the aboriginal Eskimos, and other such populations—is that #1) many members of this sect have joined it after almost a lifetime on a general or standard dietary pattern; #2) the fruits and vegetables ingested are not consciously chosen for vitamin B17 content nor are fruit seeds generally eaten by them; and #3) not all Seventh Day Adventists adhere to the vegetarian diet.

Another group that, because of religious doctrine, eats very little meat and, thus, a greater quantity of grains, vegetables, and fruits which contain B17, is the Mormon population. In Utah, which is seventy-three percent Mormon, the cancer rate is twenty-five percent below the national average. In Utah county, which includes the city of Provo and is ninety percent Mormon, the cancer rate is below the national average by twenty-eight percent for women and thirty-five percent for men.

In the summer of 1940, the Netherlands became occupied by the military forces of Nazi Germany. Under a dictatorial regime the entire nation of about nine-million people was compelled to change its eating habits drastically. Dr. C. Moerman, a physician in Vlaardingen, the Netherlands, described what happened during that period:

White bread was replaced by whole-meal bread and rye bread. The supply of sugar was drastically cut down and soon entirely stopped. Honey was used, if available. The oil supply from abroad was stopped and, as a result, no margarine was produced any more, causing the people to try and get butter. Add to this that the consumer received as much fruit and as many vegetables as possible, hoarding and buying from the farmers what they could. In short: people satisfied their hunger with large quantities of natural elements rich in vitamins.

Now think of what happened later: in 1945 this forced nutrition suddenly came to an end. What was the result? People started eating again white bread, margarine, skimmed milk, much sugar, much meat, and only few vegetables and little fruit.... In short: people ate too much unnatural and too little natural food, and therefore got too few vitamins.

Dr. Moerman showed that the cancer rate in the Netherlands dropped straight down from a peak in 1942 to its lowest point in 1945. But after 1945, with the return of processed foods, the cancer rate began to climb again and has shown a steady rise ever since.

Of course the experience in the Netherlands or among the seventh Day Adventists or Mormons is not conclusive for it still leaves open the question of the specific food factor or factors that were responsible. So let us narrow the field.

30

Since the 1960s, there has been a steadily-growing group of people who have accepted the vitamin theory of cancer and who have altered their diets accordingly. They represent all walks of life, all ages, both sexes, and reside in almost every advanced nation in the world. There are many thousands in the United States alone. It is significant, therefore, that, after maintaining a diet rich in vitamin B17, none of these people has ever been known to contract cancer.

In the summer of 1973, it was learned that Adelle Davis, one of the nation's best-known nutritionists—a woman who was considered to be an expert on the relationship between diet and cancer—herself was stricken with one of its most virulent forms. In May of the following year she passed away. It seemed that this was to be the end of the nutritional theory of cancer. But, upon closer investigation, in none of her many books or lectures did she ever treat nitrilosides as a vitamin or even as an essential food substance. She did mention that Laetrile was, in her opinion, an effective treatment for cancer after it was contracted, but she apparently failed to consider it, in its less concentrated and more natural form, as vital to one's daily nutrition. Even after her cancer had been diagnosed, she apparently still did not see the full connection. The author had corresponded with her on this very question, and her reply was, in part, as follows:

Since carcinogens surround us by the hundreds in food preservatives, additives, poison sprays, chemical fertilizers, pollutants and contaminants of air and water, the statement that cancer is a deficiency disease is certainly inaccurate and over-simplified.

It should be stated for the record that this lady was an excellent nutritionist. She had helped thousands of people regain their health through better diet and more healthful cooking. But it is plain that she did not agree with those mentioned previously who have altered their menus to include rich nitriloside foods; and so the unfortunate fact that she contracted cancer is not a disproof of the effectiveness of Laetrile.

So let us repeat the reality. While their fellow citizens are suffering from cancer at the rate of one out of every three, not one in a thousand who regularly ingests nitrilosides has been known to contract this dread disease.

For many persons, the logic of all these facts put together is so great that it would be easy to close the case right here. But, in view of the powerful opposition against this concept, let us not content ourselves with the logic of the theory. Let us reinforce our convictions with the science of the theory also, that we may understand why it works the way our logic tells us that it must.

Chapter 5

THE SEED AND THE SOIL

T. Colin Campbell, PhD, a professor at Cornell University, is the author of the most far-ranging study ever carried out on the link between cancer and dietary habits. He spent his childhood on a farm, and perhaps his knowledge of the land has been useful, because he described the relationship between diet and the development of cancer in a particularly compelling way. He compared the three stages of tumor growth—initiation, promotion, and progression—to the growth of weeds. Initiation is the phase when a seed settles in the soil. Promotion is the phase when the seed becomes a plant. Progression is the phase when the plant becomes a weed, developing beyond control, invading flower beds and garden paths, growing right up to the sidewalk. A plant that doesn't spread is not a weed.

Initiation—the presence of a potentially dangerous seed—depends largely on our genes and toxins in our environment (radiation, carcinogenic chemicals, etc.). But the seed's growth (promotion) depends on the existence of the indispensable conditions for its survival: favorable soil, water, and sun. In the book Campbell devoted to his thirty-five years of experimentation on the role of nutritional factors in cancer, he concluded: "Promotion is reversible, depending on whether the early cancer growth is given the right conditions in which to grow. This is where dietary factors are so important. These dietary factors, called promoters, feed cancer growth. Other dietary factors, called anti-promoters, slow cancer growth. Cancer flourishes when there are more promoters than anti-promoters. Cancer growth slows or

33

stops when the anti-promoters prevail. It's a push-pull process. The profound importance of this reversibility cannot be overemphasized."

Even when the nutritional conditions for maximum promotion are present—as is the case in Western diets—it is thought that fewer than one cancerous cell out of ten thousand manages to become a tumor capable of invading tissues. By acting on the soil in which these cancer seeds are deposited, it is thus possible to considerably reduce their chances of developing. This is probably what happens with Asians, who carry as many microtumors as Westerners in their bodies, but whose microtumors don't become aggressive, cancerous growths. As in an organic garden, we can learn to control weeds by controlling the mix of the soil: limiting what feeds them—the "promoters"— and abundantly supplying the nutrients that stop them from growing—"the antipromoters."

This is exactly what the great English surgeon Stephen Paget understood. In The Lancet in 1889 he published an article describing his hypothesis, which is still considered authoritative 120 years later. The name he gave it is worthy of an Aesop fable: "the seed and soil hypothesis."

A century later in the journal Nature, researchers at the Cancer Research Institute of the University of California at San Francisco showed the pertinence of that idea, and with respect to very aggressive cancer cells. If the tumor's environment is deprived of the inflammatory factors needed for its growth, it will not succeed in spreading. The fact is that these inflammatory factors, these fertilizers for cancer, are provided directly by our diet. Major dietary fertilizers are refined sugars, which drive up proinflammatory insulin and IGF; insufficient amounts of omega-3s and the corresponding excess of omega-6s, which change into inflammatory molecules; and growth hormones (present in meat and nonorganic dairy products), which also stimulate IGF. Conversely, diet may also furnish "antipromoters," such as all the phytochemical components of some vegetables or particular fruits, which directly counterbalance inflammatory mechanisms (see below).

When Richard Béliveau talks about Western diets in light of these findings, he is distressed. "With all I've learned over these years of research, if I were asked to design a diet today that promoted the development of cancer to the maximum, I couldn't improve on our present diet!"

Foods That Act Like Medications

If certain foods in our diet can act as fertilizers for tumors, others, to the contrary, harbor precious anticancer molecules. As recent discoveries show, these go far beyond the usual vitamins, minerals, and antioxidants.

In nature, when confronted with aggression, vegetables can neither fight nor flee. To survive, they must be armed with powerful molecules capable of defending them against bacteria, insects, and bad weather. These molecules are phytochemical compounds with antimicrobial, antifungal, and insecticide properties that act on the biological mechanisms of potential aggressors. They also have antioxidant properties that protect the plant's cells from dampness and the sun's rays (by preventing cellular "rust" from forming when the cell's fragile mechanisms are exposed to the corrosive effects of oxygen).

Green Tea Blocks Tissue Invasion and Angiogenesis

Green tea, for example, which grows in particularly humid climates, contains numerous polyphenols called catechins. One of these, epigallocatechin gallate or EGCG, is one of the most powerful nutritional molecules against the formation of new blood vessels by cancerous cells. It is destroyed during the fermentation required to make black tea but is found in large quantities in tea that hasn't undergone fermentation and thus remains "green." After two or three cups of green tea, EGCG is plentiful in the blood. It spreads throughout the body by means of capillary vessels. They surround and feed every cell in the body. EGCG settles on the surface of each cell and blocks the switches (the "receptors") whose function is to set off the signal that allows the penetration of neighboring tissue by foreign cells, such as cancer cells. EGCG is also capable of blocking receptors that issue commands for the creation of new vessels. Once the receptors are blocked by EGCG molecules, they no longer respond to the orders that cancer cells send through inflammation factors to invade tissue and to make the new vessels needed for tumor growth.

In their molecular medicine laboratory in Montreal, Richard Béliveau and his team tested the effects of EGCG isolated from green tea on several lines of cancer cells. They observed that it substantially slowed the growth of leukemia and breast, prostate, kidney, skin, and mouth cancer.

Green tea also acts as a detoxifier for the body. It activates mechanisms in the liver that can then eliminate cancerous toxins from the body more rapidly. In mice, it has been shown to block the effects of chemical carcinogens responsible for breast, lung, esophageal, stomach, and colon cancer.

36

Finally, the effect of EGCG is still more striking when it is combined with other molecules commonly found in Asian diets—for example, soy. The Laboratory of Nutrition and Metabolism at Harvard has shown that, when taken together, the combination of green tea and soy enhances the protective effects observed when each is taken separately. This is true for both prostate and breast cancer. In the conclusion of their article, the researchers wrote: "Our study suggests that soy phytochemicals plus green tea may be used as a potentially effective dietary regimen for inhibiting progression of estrogen dependent breast cancer." In the extremely cautious language that characterizes scientific articles on cancer (not to mention the reserved style of Harvard researchers) these words are highly significant.

How Many Cups of Green Tea Per Day?

This question is answered by two studies on patients in Japan, a country full of green tea drinkers. In a group of Japanese women suffering from breast tumors that had not yet metastasized, researchers discovered that those who consumed three cups of green tea a day had 57 percent * fewer relapses than those who only drank one cup a day. In men with prostate tumors, daily consumption of five cups of green tea reduced the risk that their cancer would progress to an advanced stage by 50 percent. The effect of green tea is quite remarkable. So why deprive ourselves?

Is Olive Oil the Green Tea of the Mediterranean Diet?

Everyone has heard of the beneficial effects of the "Mediterranean diet." Epidemiological studies have shown that people who follow a Mediterranean diet are, on average, far less affected by degenerative illness, cardiac disease, and cancer, despite the significant

37

presence of fats in their diet. For a long time, the benefits of this diet were attributed to its combination of fiber, fish, fruit, and vegetables whose antioxidant potential and wealth of anticancer phytochemical agents have been demonstrated. Recently, researchers have realized that a determining factor in the etiology of some cancers is not only the quantity, but also the type of fats consumed. It's now time to pay closer attention to a central ingredient in Mediterranean cooking: olives, and the oil that we extract from them.

A study directed by Dr. Robert Owen of the German Cancer Research Center in Heidelberg has demonstrated that olives contain an abundance of antioxidants such as acteosides, hydroxytyrosol, tyrosol, and phenylpropionic acids. The direct effect of such molecules is to limit the initial development of cancer.

Particularly when it is virgin, olive oil also contains secoiridoids and lignans, both known antioxidants that have been linked with slower progression of cancer.

Since all these chemicals are fat soluble, they are absorbed into fatty tissues, with a resulting known protective effect against breast cancer, colon cancer, and uterine cancer.

At the Catalan Oncology Institute, another group of researchers analyzed the effects of chemical agents contained in olive oil on certain genes. These Spanish researchers demonstrated that polyphenols and oleic acid can inhibit expression of the HER2 gene, which has been implicated in close to one fifth of breast cancers. The researchers emphasize, however, that to obtain this result, we would have to ingest olive oil in quantities difficult to achieve through normal consumption. I do not recommend using olive oil to replace Herceptin, a medication that is very effective in inhibiting the HER2 gene. On the other hand, I do recommend olive oil as part of a daily diet because continuous consumption over the course of months or years may have a small daily effect on these genes. In synergy with all the other foods in the Mediterranean diet, olive oil may contribute to slowing the progression of cancer. It is also possible that consumption of olive oil by women taking Herceptin may increase the efficacy of the medication.

Soy Blocks Dangerous Hormones

Soy, too, contains powerful phytochemical molecules that counteract the mechanisms essential to the survival and spread of cancer. These are the soy isoflavones—especially genistein, daidzein, and glycitein. They are called phytoestrogens because they are very similar to female estrogens. The abundance of natural and chemical estrogens in Western women is known to be one of the causes of the breast cancer epidemic. This is why today hormone replacement therapy is prescribed to postmenopausal women only with great caution: It is associated with an increased risk of breast cancer. Soy phytoestrogens are only one hundredth as biologically active as natural female estrogens. They act along the same lines as tamoxifen—a drug commonly used to prevent relapses in breast cancer. Their presence in the blood substantially lowers overstimulation of the body by estrogens and, as a consequence, may slow the growth of estrogen-dependent tumors. However, the protective action of soy against breast cancer has been formally demonstrated only for women who have consumed it since adolescence. Its protective effect against cancer has not been proven where consumption begins in adulthood. As one of the soy isoflavones, genistein, closely resembles male hormones that stimulate the growth of prostate cancers, the same protective mechanism is likewise at work in men who consume soy regularly.

Moreover, like EGCG in green tea, soy isoflavones also block angiogenesis. They thus play an important role in fighting a number of other cancers besides breast and prostate cancer. Different forms of soy (tofu, tempeh, miso, edamame, etc.) are therefore likely to be a useful part of an anticancer diet.

Berries: Blackberries, Raspberries, Strawberries, Blueberries . . .

In its fight against cancer, the pharmaceutical industry is also actively pursuing leads to antiangiogenic drugs. Richard Béliveau has also worked since the midnineties on antiangiogenic medications that the industry has asked him to test in his laboratory. His work consists of growing in vitro blood vessel cells stimulated by chemical growth "boosters" like those made by cancerous tumors. With a micropipette, a tiny dose of the test medication is applied to the boosted cells to measure their capacity to prevent the creation of new blood vessels. It takes several days before any effects, often relatively subtle, can be detected.

Béliveau remembers mornings when he arrived in his laboratory, impatient to find out if this or that new molecule had passed the test. Any time he observed a promising effect, his adrenaline would rise and he would call the pharmaceutical firm with a triumphant "We've got a hit!" These promising results would galvanize the firm to invest even more money in the work, and Dr. Béliveau would quickly find himself heading a large-scale research program. However, there was always a shadow over this rosy picture. In this type of research, 95 percent of these promising synthetic molecules end up rejected when they are evaluated on animals and then on humans. Even when they are effective against cancer cells in a test tube, they are usually too toxic to be prescribed. But today, in the laboratory of molecular medicine of the Sainte-Justine Children's Hospital, the atmosphere is no longer quite the same.

Instead of evaluating a new chemical molecule, Béliveau recently decided to examine the antiangiogenic potential of an extract of raspberry. Ellagic acid is a polyphenol found in large quantities in raspberries and strawberries (it is also found in hazelnuts and walnuts). In doses amounting to a normal dietary portion of raspberries or strawberries, ellagic acid had already shown it could slow tumor growth significantly in mice exposed to aggressive carcinogens.

Tested with the same rigor as that applied to any drug, Béliveau found, ellagic acid in raspberries is potentially just as effective as a medication proven to slow the growth of blood vessels. Indeed, ellagic acid was shown to act against the two most common mechanisms of stimulation of blood vessels (vascular endothelial growth factor, or VEGF, and platelet-derived growth factor, or PDGF). Béliveau knew how important this discovery was. If it had been a pharmaceutical molecule, his fax machine would have been going all day and the grants would have poured in. All the more so in this case, then, since there was no risk of discovering later that the promising molecule was too toxic for use on humans: After all, hominids have been eating raspberries since prehistoric times. But whom should he call? There was no question of a patent on raspberries; thus, there was nobody on the other end of the line to share the excitement of the moment and no grant money to be won.

Small fruits such as strawberries and raspberries (or walnuts, hazelnuts, and pecans) are more promising still. Unlike classic antiangiogenic drugs, their action is not confined to this single mechanism. Ellagic acid also detoxifies cells: It blocks the transformation of environmental carcinogens into toxic substances and stimulates the elimination of toxins. The toxins we are referring to here are dangerous because they interact with DNA and provoke potentially life-threatening genetic mutations. Hence, ellagic acid is a kind of supermolecule that acts on several fronts, and without side effects.

Another natural anticancer food is cherries, which contain glucaric acid, a substance that can detoxify the body by facilitating elimination of the xenoestrogens that come from environmental chemicals. Blueberries contain anthocyanidins and proanthocyanidins, molecules that are capable of forcing cancer cells to commit suicide (apoptosis). In the laboratory, these molecules act on several cancer lines and are particularly effective against colon cancer. Other rich sources of proanthocyanidins are cranberries, cinnamon, and dark chocolate.

Recent studies in animals have confirmed these laboratory results. Researchers at Ohio State University showed that rats who consumed black raspberries from Canada experienced an inhibiting effect on cancers of the esophagus, mouth, and colon. A team led by Professor Gary Stoner obtained equivalent results with raspberry powder containing a high concentration of anthocyanins. In both cases, rats in the group that consumed the berries developed 50 percent fewer tumors than the control group. This magical little fruit has already proven its effects in a small group of patients who genetically suffer from a particular kind of polyp that is known to aggravate the risk of breast cancer. Patients who took black raspberry extract had up to 59 percent fewer of these dangerous polyps than the group who were given a placebo.

Plums, Peaches, and Nectarines: It's Time for Stone Fruit

Berries have recently found some competition: peaches, plums, nectarines, etc. (collectively known as stone fruit), whose anticancer virtues were previously unknown. According to a group of researchers in Texas who reviewed more than a hundred species, these fruits—particularly plums—are at least as rich in anticancer elements as small berries. In this time of economic recession, it's good to know that a single plum contains as many antioxidants as a handful of berries and costs far less. In laboratory tests, stone fruits have also demonstrated their efficacy against breast cancer cells and cholesterol.

Spices and Herbs Acting on the Same Mechanisms as Medications

In 2001 the Food and Drug Administration broke all speed records in approving a new anticancer drug—Gleevec. This medication is effective in treating both a common form of leukemia and a very rare and typically fatal intestinal cancer. In an enthusiastic interview in the New York Times, Dr. Larry Norton, the former president of the American Society for Clinical Oncology and one of the principal oncologists at Memorial Sloan-Kettering

Hospital in New York, did not mince his words. He called Gleevec's effects "a miracle."

Indeed, to oncologists, Gleevec has inaugurated an entirely novel approach to treating cancer. Rather than trying to poison cancer cells (as chemotherapy does), Gleevec blocks the cellular mechanisms that day after day enable the cancer to grow. It acts on one of the genes that stimulate cancer growth, but it is now thought that another key function may be to block one of the switches that stimulate the creation of new blood vessels (the PDGF receptor). Administered daily, Gleevec can "contain" cancer growth, which then ceases to be dangerous. We have reached the stage of "cancer without disease," in the language of Judah Folkman, who discovered angiogenesis.

It so happens that many herbs and spices act along some of the same lines as Gleevec. This is true of the labiate family, for example, which includes mint, thyme, marjoram, oregano, basil, and rosemary. They are rich in fatty acids of the terpene family, which makes them particularly fragrant. Terpenes have been shown to act on a wide variety of tumors by reducing the spread of cancer cells or by provoking their death.

One of these terpenes—carnosol in rosemary—affects the capacity of cancer cells to invade neighboring tissues. When it is incapable of spreading, cancer loses its virulence. Moreover, researchers at the National Cancer Institute have demonstrated that rosemary extracts help chemotherapy penetrate cancer cells. In tissue cultures, they lower the resistance of breast cancer cells to chemotherapy.

In Richard Béliveau's experiments, apigenine—plentiful in parsley and celery—has demonstrated powerful

44

inhibition of the creation of blood vessels, which tumors need to grow, and to a degree comparable to Gleevec. This effect occurs even with very small concentrations, similar to those observed in the blood after consumption of parsley.

HEALTHY DIET AND CANCER – THE MISSING LINK

While dealing with cancer, most of us ignore the importance of a healthy diet. Latest research shows that there is a strong connection between the quality of food we eat and the likelihood of developing cancer. If we take the right food, it will greatly increase the odds of beating cancer. Mother Nature offers us variety of healthy food items capable of fighting cancer and boosting our immune system. Some of the super heroes are listed as under:

- Cruciferous Vegetables

Some of the vegetables belonging to the Cruciferae family are considered to be the most powerful caner fighting foods. Vegetables such as Kale, Broccoli, Cabbage, Brussels, Cauliflower, and sprouts are included in this list and contain huge amounts of vitamins, fiber, minerals and antioxidants such as beta carotene, which help in boosting our immune system. Due to the presence of phytochemicals, such as isothiocyanates, these vegetables help in breaking down the potential carcinogens. Some other examples of Cruciferous vegetables are mustard greens, collard greens, rutabagas, bok choy, radish, daikon, and turnips. If you want to outsmart cancer, you need to make sure to include these vegetables in your daily diet plan.

- Turmeric

An active compound present in Turmeric known as Curcumin, has shown remarkable results when it comes to fighting cancer. Some of the latest research reveals that this active compound helps in preventing lung cancer in tobacco smokers. It is readily available in the market and is used in most of the Asian (sub continent) dishes.

- Mushrooms

We all have heard and tasted mushrooms in our lives, however there are only a few of us who know anything about the "Medical Mushrooms". Medical mushrooms are special kind of mushrooms which have the ability to fight cancer cells. They are rich in immune boosting compounds such as polysaccharides. It is because of the presence of thioproline, lentinan, lectin and beta glucan that these mushrooms are termed as the medical mushrooms. They help boost the production of interferon, which helps in preventing the cancer cells to grow and multiply.

If you are interested in trying these Medical mushrooms out, you can find them in the market by the name, cordyceps oglossoides, agaricus blazei, coriolus versicolor, reishi, and phellinus linteusf.

- Garlic

There is no better food that fights cancer like garlic does. An immune boosting compound present in garlic is known as allium, which helps in breaking down cancer causing substances and boost body's natural immune system. The allium can also be found in onions, chives and leeks; therefore all of these vegetables help in lowering the risk of colon and stomach cancer. An active ingredient in the garlic oil, which is known as diallyl sulfide has shown great results in incapacitating carcinogens in the liver.

- Hot Peppers

Hot peppers are not only hot in their taste; they are also hot in cancer treatment. They contain a chemical called capsaicin, which helps neutralize certain cancer causing cells. Jalapenos and chili peppers are especially valuable for preventing stomach cancer.

- Dark Red Grapes

Dark red grapes contain high doses of bioflavonoid, a strong antioxidant, which is known as an effective cancer preventer. Not only that, other chemicals such as resveratrol and ellagic acid help in slowing down the tumor growth by blocking the enzymes needed by the cancer cells. Most of the scientist and researchers, therefore suggest eating them full, with seeds and the skin.

- Brown Seaweed

An active compound present in the brown seaweed (Kombu) known as fucoidan (a polysaccharide) is effective in killing caner tumors. It has also shown remarkable results in treating stomach cancer and colon cancer. No doubt, the people of Okinawa in Japan, who consume Kombu in their daily food have the lowest cancer deaths and enjoy the highest life expectancies.

- Miscellaneous

Besides the above mentioned diet items, there are many other powerful cancer fighting foods within your reach, you can include them in your daily food to decrease the odds of developing any kind of cancer.

- ✓ Sweet potatoes
- ✓ Blueberries
- ✓ Extra virgin olive oil
- ✓ Carrots
- ✓ Avocados
- ✓ Tomatoes
- ✓ Raspberries
- ✓ Green Tea
- ✓ Black Tea
- ✓ Nuts
- ✓ Apples

Intermittent Fasting

Many people do it for cultural and religious purposes, but fasting has a place in cancer treatment as well—and I'm not even talking about having to starve yourself for days at a time in order to see results. Simply adjusting the times at which you eat, a protocol known as intermittent fasting, can make all the difference in getting your metabolism back on track.

It's something they do down at the Hope4Cancer Clinic in Tijuana as an adjunct to the other treatments offered there. Dialing down the time frames in which patients eat from the typical morning, noon, and night routine, which can span upwards of 12 hours or even longer, to a much smaller 6- to 8-hour window during the middle of the day has helped many people conquer their cancers faster and with greater comfort throughout the process.

Intermittent fasting has been shown to help boost insulin sensitivity and reduce insulin resistance, while at the same time promoting normalized autophagy. Oscar Puig, a nutritionist at the Hope4Cancer Institute, is keen on the "Leangains" Method of intermittent fasting, which restricts eating times to between noon and 8 P.M. every day. This method is both effective and easy to follow because the daily schedule remains the same rather than changing.

You wouldn't think that depriving a person's body of nutrition during certain hours of the day would have much effect on his cancer state, but it does. A 2009 study out of the University of Southern California found that cells respond to this period of being in "starvation mode" differently depending on whether they're healthy or malignant.

Healthy cells generally wait out this "lean period" by going into a type of hibernation mode, which protects them from damage. But cancer cells continue to grow because their genetic pathways are stuck in "on" mode, which makes them less resistant to stress and more prone to failure.

"The cell is, in fact, committing cellular suicide," stated Valter Longo, an associate professor of gerontology and biology at the University of Southern California, who for years has been studying the effects of intermittent fasting on cancer and how cancer cells respond to this nontoxic therapy. "What we're seeing is that the cancer cell tries to compensate for the lack of all these things missing in the blood after fasting. It may be trying to replace them, but it can't."

The fact of the matter is that every type of cancer is treatable with metabolic therapy, whether it involves intermittent fasting, R-KD, enzyme therapy, or some combination of all of these. As Professor Seyfried puts it, all types of cancer have "the same, beautiful, metabolic target" painted on their backs, which means beating this dreadful disease is simply a matter of hitting it, and hitting it hard.

What You Need To Know

- The human body is designed to efficiently remove dead cells and waste as it constantly regenerates new healthy cells (autophagy), but excess toxins and nutrient deficiency can impede this important process.

- Emerging research shows that enzyme therapy can help restore autophagy and reverse the health conditions caused by its breakdown.

- Metabolic therapies that utilize enzymes, detoxification, and diet are proving to be even more effective at restoring autophagy.

- Comprehensive immunotherapeutic protocols like those offered at the Issels Clinic utilize enzymes, oxygen, energy, detoxification, homeopathy, nutrition, and more to restore optimal health.

- Supplementing daily with proteolytic enzymes is a great way to prevent autophagic breakdown and the formation of chronic illness.

- Teaching your body to rely on fats rather than carbohydrates for energy (restricted ketogenic diet) can help starve cancer cells.

- Intermittent fasting can also help promote a normalized state of autophagy.

ENZYMES

"Climb the mountains and get their good tidings. Nature's peace will flow into you as sunshine flows into trees. The winds will blow their own freshness into you, and the storms their energy, while cares will drop off like autumn leaves." John Muir, co-founder of national parks.

Enzymes are organic catalysts that speed up the rate of a chemical reaction. In simple terms, enzymes in the body either "glue" stuff together (called conjugase) or tear stuff apart (called hydrolase). Without enzymes, life on earth could not exist. Enzymes wear out and are still a great source of mystery to leading researchers.

In the 1920s, scientists in Germany found that cancer patients seemed to lack a factor in the blood. They began injecting animal tumors with pineapple juice extract, which contains the proteolytic enzyme bromelain, and watched a measurable shrinkage or disappearance of many cancers in animals.

There are impressive studies showing that certain enzymes when taken orally as pills can reduce the toxicity of chemo and radiation, while extending the quality and quantity of life for most cancer patients. The German FDA has approved the use of injectable forms of enzymes, which are 100 times more potent than taking oral enzymes which must pass through the gut into the bloodstream. Enzymes taken in fairly large quantities on an empty stomach will be partially absorbed into the blood stream and may help fight the cancer. Enzymes taken with a meal will help digest the food in that meal, but probably will not be absorbed into the bloodstream to fight the cancer.

There are literally millions of enzymes produced by your body each second. Without hydrolase enzymes in your gut, the digestion of food could not occur. Our body makes digestive enzymes to break down large food particles into usable molecules:

- proteins are digested into amino acids by the action of proteases, including trypsin and chymotrypsin

- starches are digested into simple sugars by the action of amylase

- fats are digested into fatty acids and glycerol by the action of lipase.

Our ancestors ate a diet high in uncooked foods. Cooking food denatures enzymes, like changing the white on an egg from waxey to white when it is cooked. It makes no difference whether you cook the food over a fire, on the barbeque, in the microwave oven, or fry it on the stovetop...all forms of heat denature enzymes. All living tissue contains an abundance of hydrolase enzymes as part of the lysosomes, or "suicide bags", which are there to mop up cellular debris and destroy invading organisms. When our ancestors ate this diet high in uncooked food, they were receiving a regular infusion of "enzyme therapy" as a lucky by-product. These hydrolytic enzymes would help to digest the food, and about 10% of the unused enzymes would end up crossing through the intestinal wall into the blood stream.

It is clear that people who are undernourished without being malnourished live a longer and healthier life. Why this occurs is less obvious. Many good European studies support the use of digestive enzymes as a critical component of cancer treatment. Your mouth, stomach, and intestines will make a certain amount of enzymes to digest your food into smaller molecules for absorption through the intestinal wall into the bloodstream. Enzymes absorbed into the bloodstream help to break up immune complexes, expose tumors to immune attack, and assist in cell differentiation. People who eat less food may live longer because they are able to absorb a certain percentage of their unused digestive enzymes, which then have many therapeutic benefits. Indeed, as far back as 1934, an Austrian researcher, Dr. E. Freund, found that cancer patients do not have the "solubilizing" tumor-destroying enzymes in their blood that normal healthy people have.

The vast majority of cancer patients are older people, who have demonstrated a reduced output of digestive enzymes. Raw foods, which are high in hydrolytic enzymes, may sometimes help cancer patients.

There are 30 years of good research from Europe showing that enzyme therapy may help cancer patients. Digestive enzymes can:

♦ reduce tumor growth and metastasis in experimental animals.

♦ prevent radon-induced lung cancer in miners.

♦ improve 5 year survival in breast cancer patients. Stage I at 91%, stage II at 75%, and stage III at 50%.

♦ bromelain (enzyme from pineapple) inhibited leukemic cell growth and induced human leukemia cells in culture to revert back to normal (cytodifferentiation).

♦ reduce the complications of cancer, such as cachexia (weight loss), pain in joints, and depression.

♦ reduced the secondary infections that result from certain chemo and radiation methods, especially bleomycin-induced pneumotoxicity.

Proteolytic enzymes (proteases), such as bromelain from pineapple, seem to dissolve the "stealth" coating that keeps tumors invisible from the cancer patient's "radar". Proteases also break up "circulating immune complexes", which makes the immune system more efficient against cancer. Proteases have recently been found to be part of the body's complex regulation and communication system, possibly helping to induce apoptosis (suicide) in cancer cells. Best food sources of these proteolytic enzymes are pineapple, papaya, mango, and kiwi.

Wobenzym is a unique clinically-tested product from Germany with a proprietary blend of various plant and animal-derived digestive enzymes, coupled with rutin (a bioflavonoid) all packaged in an enterically coated pill to survive the acid bath of the stomach and move into the intestines for absorption.

Serrapeptase (technically Serrato Peptidase) is a proteolytic enzyme produced by bacteria in the gut of silkworms. Serrapeptase has been studied and used extensively in Europe and Asia for over a quarter century, and seems to reduce swelling and digest unnecessary fibrin in the body. In one study, 70 women with fibrocystic breast disease were randomly divided into either treatment with serrapeptase or placebo group. The serrapeptase group had a greater reduction in breast swelling and pain than the placebo group.

Enzymes are measured in USP (United States Pharmacopeia) comparison to pancreatic extract. One of the functions of the pancreas is to make digestive enzymes. A 4x label on your enzymes means "4 times the potency of pancreatin USP". Therefore, 500 mg of 4X pancreatin is equal in digestive capacity to 2,000 mg of pancreatin USP. 50,000 USP units is a good target for any given meal or in between meal dosage.

Enzymes taken with a meal will help to digest the food, but will not be absorbed into the bloodstream to help fight the cancer. About 10% of enzymes taken on an empty stomach will be absorbed into the bloodstream to help fight the cancer. Enzymes are one of the more fragile molecules in nature, easily denatured by temperatures above 108 F.

Along with iron, vitamin A is one of the most common micronutrient deficiencies in the world. Around the world, an estimated 500,000 people each year go permanently blind because of clinical vitamin A deficiency. Vitamin A was the first micronutrient to be recognized for its role in preventing cancer. Vitamin A is one of the most multi-talented of all substances in human nutrition and plays a key role in preventing and reversing cancer. While vitamin A and beta-carotene are considered interchangeable, more recent evidence shows that these two nutrients have some overlapping functions and some distinctly different functions. A drug analog of vitamin A (all trans retinoic acid) has become a near cure all for acute promyelocytic leukemia, with one study showing a 96% cure rate. 2 Some companies use an emulsified vitamin A so that it stays in the blood stream longer, which may be important for extremely high doses of A (>100,000 iu/day) in cancer patients.

All of the known functions of vitamin A relate either directly or indirectly to the cancer patient:

♦ Cell division. Billions of times each day, cells divide in the precarious process of cell division, i.e. proliferation or hyperplasia. Without vitamin A, this fragile process can easily turn into cancer, or neoplasia. Vitamin A is crucial for cancer prevention. Vitamin A deficiency may be one of the primary insults leading to lung cancer. There are probably binding sites on the human DNA for vitamin A. Researchers found that one of the most common cancers in Third World countries, cervical cancer, was linked to Human Papilloma Virus, which was then linked to shutting off the cancer-protective gene, called p53, which was then linked to a low intake of vitamin A. Essentially, vitamin A keeps the p53 active and protecting our DNA against cancer, even from viral attack.

♦ Cell-to-cell communication, a.k.a. gap junction. Cells communicate via a "telegraph" system of ions floating in and out of cell membrane pores. This intercellular communication helps to maintain cooperation and coordination of cell functions. Without vitamin A, the "telegraph" system becomes distorted, and cancer can arise.

♦ Maintenance of epithelial tissue, or skin. The vast majority of cancers, including lung, breast, colon, and prostate, all arise from the epithelial tissue and are called carcinomas. Other categories of cancers include: leukemia (cancer of the bone marrow that produces red & white cells), lymphoma (cancer of the lymph cells and glands), and sarcomas (cancers of the structural tissue). When the body is deprived of vitamin A, skin (epithelial) cancer is more likely to result. Giving therapeutic doses of vitamin A has been shown to slow down and reverse some forms of cancer.

♦ Immune stimulant. Vitamin A deficiency brings changes in the mucosal membranes, changes in lymphocyte sub-populations, and altered T- and B-cell functions. There are many studies linking vitamin A supplements to the curing of measles. Vitamin A supplements brought a 19% reduction in respiratory infections in children. HIV-positive pregnant women with the lowest quartile of serum vitamin A had a 400% increase in the risk of transmitting their HIV virus to their unborn infant.

♦ Anti-cancer activity. Vitamin A supplements as sole therapy in patients with unresectable (canno be surgically removed) lung cancer measurably improved immune functions and tumor response. Vitamin A, and not beta-carotene, improved lymphocyte levels and reduced complications after surgery in lung cancer patients. In patients treated for bladder cancer, the incidence of recurrence was 180% higher in patients who consumed the lowest quartile of vitamin A in the diet. High doses of vitamin A (200,000 iu/week) were able to reduce damaged and potentially cancerous mouth cells by 96%. Vitamin A and its synthetic analogues have been shown to improve cancer treatment in oral leukoplakia, laryngeal papillomatosis, superficial bladder carcinoma, cervical dysplasia, bronchial metaplasia, and preleukemia. Vitamin A supplements of 300,000 iu per day were provided in a placebo-controlled trial with 307 patients with stage I non-small-cell lung cancer. 37% of the treated group experienced a recurrence, while 48% of the non-treated group had a recurrence, thus bringing a 25% reduction in tumor recurrence, when used as the sole therapy.

SAFETY ISSUES. While vitamins, in general, are much safer than drugs, it is important to discuss vitamin A toxicity, which is by far the most common cause of vitamin toxicity. Up to 1 million iu of vitamin A per day has been given for 5 years without side effects in European cancer clinics. One study found that women taking as little as 10,000 iu/day during pregnancy had a slightly elevated risk for having a child with birth defects (teratogenicity). Another study from the National Institutes of Health found no increase in birth defects in women taking 25,000 iu/day of vitamin A. An FDA biochemist, John Hathcock, PhD, states that toxicity with vitamin A at these low levels mainly involves people with confounding medical conditions, including compromised liver function.

Cancer clinics in Europe often administer up to 2.5 million iu/day of vitamin A in emulsified form for several months under medical supervision. While these doses are not recommended without medical supervision, it shows the relative safety of vitamin A in the general population. Giving at least 300,000 iu per day of retinol palmitate in 138 lung cancer patients for at least 12 months created self- terminating unremarkable symptoms in less than 10% of these patients and only caused interruption of treatment in 3% due to symptoms that were potentially related to vitamin A excess. Upset stomach (dyspepsia), headache, nosebleeds, and mild hair loss were the most common and self-limiting symptoms.

Since primitive meat-eating populations would usually eat the liver of the animal first, which is the most concentrated source of pre-formed vitamin A, descendants of carnivorous people probably have a much greater tolerance and need for higher doses of A. By increasing the intake of vitamin E, many people will be able to avoid toxicity from high doses of vitamin A, since it is the lipid peroxide products from A that can cause damage to the liver. Vitamin E prevents lipid peroxidation.

PREGNANT WOMEN SHOULD NOT USE HIGH DOSES OF VITAMIN A.

It is easy to appreciate the beauty of carotenoids on a crisp, fall day with the autumn foliage at its peak. Carotenoids are usually pigmented substances produced by plants to assist in photosynthesis and to protect the plant from the damaging effects of the sun's radiation. Of the 800 or so carotenoids that have been isolated, the most famous are beta-carotene, alpha-carotene, lutein, zeaxanthin, lycopene, and beta-cryptoxanthin. Most carotenoids are pigmented molecules that are red, yellow, or orange in color. A few carotenoids, such as phytoene and phytofluene, are colorless.

Over 200 epidemiological studies 19 show that a diet rich in fruit and vegetables will lower the risk for a variety of cancers. Of the 15% of annual lung cancer patients who are not smokers, which totals over 22,000 deaths per year, fruits and vegetables can provide major protection against lung cancer.

Beta-carotene and other carotenoids have been thoroughly reviewed regarding their role in cancer and it has been found: "...carotenoids exert an important influence in modulating the actions of carcinogens." Beta-carotene has been shown to play a major role in the "telegraph"-like communication between cells that prevents or reverses abnormal growths. This "gap junction communication" is one of many reasons why beta-carotene protects us from cancer. Beta-carotene selectively inhibited the growth of human squamous cancer cells in culture. Beta-carotene and canthaxanthin provided significant protection in animals against the cancer-causing effects of radiation.

Carotenoids may partially compensate for the "sins" of our unhealthy lifestyles. In one study, researchers from the National Cancer Institute and Harvard tracked over 47,000 healthy individuals and found that lycopenes, even from pizza sauce, were protective against prostate cancer. Other studies have found that beta-carotene supplements can reverse the pre-cancerous condition (oral leukoplakia) brought about by chewing betel nut, 26 which is a Third World version of chewing tobacco.

Beta-carotene affects the cancer process in a variety of ways:

♦ alters the adenylate cyclase activity in melanoma cells in culture, which affects cell differentiation and, thus, whether a cell will turn cancerous or not

♦ potent anti-oxidant, which spares immune cells in the microscopic "war on cancer" and protects the healthy prostaglandins

♦ provides a certain level of tumor immunity in mice inoculated with cancer cells

♦ protects the DNA against the damaging effects of carcinogens

♦ according to studies by Food and Drug Administration researchers, beta-carotene protects against the cancer causing effects of a choline deficient diet in animals

♦ once cancer has been initiated, either chemically or physically, beta-carotene inhibits the next step in the cancer process of neoplastic transformation

♦ there is a synergistic benefit of using vitamin A with carotenoids in patients who have been first treated with chemo, radiation, and surgery for common malignancies

♦ beta-carotene and vitamin A together provided a significant improvement in outcome in animals treated with radiation for induced cancers

♦ carotenoids (from Spirulina and Dunaliella algae) plus vitamin E and canthaxanthin were injected in animal tumors, with the result being complete regression, as mediated by an increase in Tumor Necrosis Factor (TNF) in macrophages in the tumor region

♦ in 20 patients with mouth cancer who were given high doses of radiation and chemo, beta-carotene provided significant protection against mouth sores (oral mucositis) induced by medical therapy, although there was no significant difference in survival rates

♦ in animals, beta-carotene provided cancer protection against a carcinogenic virus, which would normally damage the DNA

Betatene is a special, mixed carotenoid extract from Dunaliella algae that has been shown in scientific studies to potently inhibit the development of breast tumors in animals. Betatene consists of a rich mixture of various carotenoids, primarily naturally-occurring betacarotene, along with smaller amounts of lycopene, alpha-carotene, zeaxanthin, cryptoxanthin, and lutein.

NUTRITIONAL SYNERGISM

Zinc deficiency in animals further compounds a vitamin E deficiency, meaning that zinc must be present to properly utilize vitamin E. Also, vitamin E protects the body against the potentially damaging effects of iron and rusting fish oil. Human volunteers given high doses of fish oil experienced an immune abnormality (mitogenic responsiveness of peripheral blood mononuclear cells to concanavalin A), which was reversed with supplements of vitamin E.

IMMUNE REGULATOR

Vitamin E plays a powerful role as an immune regulator. When 32 healthy elderly adults were given supplements of 800 iu daily of vitamin E, there were measurable improvements in immune functions. Following 28 days of supplements of vitamins E, C, and A researchers found that 30 elderly institutionalized patients had substantial improvements in immune functions (absolute T-cells, T4 subsets, T4:T8 ratio, and lymphocyte proliferation). E seems to work by protecting immune factors from immediate destruction in their suicidal plunge at cancer cells. E also works by bolstering the activity of the thymus and spleen organs to stimulate lymphocyte proliferation. In burned animals, vitamin E supplements offered substantial protection in the intestinal mucosa to prevent bacterial translocation (gut bacteria migrating into the blood to cause septicemia).

PROTECTION FROM TOXINS

Vitamin E protected animals from the cancer-causing effects of alcohol on the esophagus and a carcinogen on the colon. Vitamin E and selenium protected animals against the potent carcinogenic effects of DMBA from tobacco. Vitamin E protected the damaged liver of rats from developing fatty liver and collagen content. Vitamin E protects us against the greatest toxin and essential nutrient of them all--oxygen, as shown in exercised animals. 72 By

sparing fats in the blood from becoming lipid peroxides, vitamin E supplements were very effective at preventing heart disease. Vitamin E prevents the formation of one of the more common carcinogenic agents in humans--nitrosamines--which are formed by the combination of nitrates in the diet and amino acids in the stomach.

Vitamin E prevents damage to the skin from ultraviolet radiation. According to researchers from Bulgaria, vitamin E protects us against the harmful effects of too many iron-generating free radicals and damage to our detoxification system, cytochrome P-450.

Much of the damage caused by iron in the human body is due to:

1) wrong form of iron, we need chelated iron, not iron salts as we get in fortified white flour

2) not enough antioxidants to prevent this oxidizing metal from "rusting" in the cell and creating harm.

3) lowering of pH, or acidosis, which causes iron to become unbound from its protective shells of hemoglobin and transferrin

REVERSE PRE-CANCEROUS CONDITION
Vitamin E supplements (200-400 mg/d for 3 months) reversed fibrocystic breast disease (a major risk for breast cancer) in 22 out of 26 women. Other women have found reversal of fibrocystic breast disease through elimination of caffeine, chocolate, and colas, which contain methylxanthines.

PROSTAGLANDINS
We can generate very healthy prostaglandins, if we have the right dietary precursors in our blood, which come from:

♦ enough fish oil (EPA) or flax oil (ALA) and borage oil (GLA)

♦ healthy levels of blood sugar (60-100 mg%)

♦ optimal amounts of vitamin E

Because of this beneficial impact on prostaglandins, vitamin E helps to inhibit platelet adhesion, which helps to slow down the spreading of cancer. And yet, as shown below, vitamin E does not influence blood clotting, or prothrombin time, which is good news for people worried about proper clotting during and after surgery.

SLOWS AND REVERSES CANCER

In human studies, low intake of vitamin E increases the risk for cancer of various body sites. Patients with head and neck cancers are more likely to have a recurrence if they have low blood levels of vitamins E, A, and beta-carotene. Vitamin E injected into animal mouth tumors was able to significantly reduce or completely eliminate tumors. 80 In

patients with colorectal cancer, vitamin E, C, and A supplements were able to reduce the growth of abnormal cells in the colon, indicating a possible slowing of the cancer process. In human epidemiology studies, people with the highest intake of E (still very low compared to ideal intake) had a 40% reduction in the risk for colon cancer. 82 In animals, vitamin E supplements prevent lung tumors from developing.

VITAMIN E SUCCINATE AND CANCER

When vitamin E is esterified (combined) with succinic acid, a new molecule is formed with surprising ability to selectively shut down cancer growth, but not harm healthy tissue, slowing the growth of brain (glioma and neuroblastoma) and melanoma cells in culture. E succinate is able to reduce the genetic expression of c-myc oncogenes in cultured cancer cells. E succinate inhibits virally-induced tumors in culture. E succinate has been studied as a potent regulator of cell proliferation.

IMPROVES MEDICAL THERAPY OF CANCER

Vitamin E helps generally toxic medical therapies to distinguish between healthy and cancerous cells. The best proposed mechanism for this action is the anaerobic state of many tumors. Vitamin E apparently is not well absorbed, or needed, by tumors, since they are anaerobic (without oxygen). An antioxidant is of little interest to an oxygen- independent cell. Because of this function of vitamin E, chemotherapy and radiation can be made much more selectively toxic to the cancer cells, while protecting the patient from host damage.

It has long been known that a vitamin E deficiency, common in cancer patients, will accentuate the cardiotoxic effects of adriamycin. The worse the vitamin E deficiency in animals, the greater the heart damage from adriamycin. Patients undergoing chemo, radiation, and bone marrow transplant for cancer treatment had markedly depressed levels of serum antioxidants, including vitamin E. Given the fact that both chemo and radiation can induce cancer, which reduces the chances for survival, it is noteworthy that vitamin E protects animals against a potent carcinogen, DMBA. Vitamin E supplements prevented the glucose-raising effects of a chemo drug, doxorubicin. Since cancer is a sugar-feeder, preventing this glucose-raising effect may be another valuable contribution from vitamin E in patients receiving chemo. Meanwhile, vitamin E improves the tumor kill rate of doxorubicin. Vitamin E modifies the carcinogenic effect of daunomycin (chemo drug) in animals.

Human prostate cancer cells were killed at a higher rate when adriamycin (chemo drug) was combined with vitamin E at concentrations that can easily be obtained from supplementation. Vitamin E supplements (1,600 iu/day) taken one week prior to adriamycin therapy protected 69% of patients from hair loss, which is nearly universal in adriamycin-treated patients. Vitamin E helped to repair kidney damage caused by adriamycin in animals. Vitamin E and selenium supplements in animals helped to reduce the heart toxicity from adriamycin. Selenium and vitamin E supplements

were given to 41 women undergoing cytotoxic therapy for ovarian and cervical cancers, with a resulting drop in the toxicity-related rise in creatine kinase. Vitamin E, A, and prenylamine reduced the toxicity of adriamycin on the hearts of animals studied.

In animals with implanted tumors, those pretreated with vitamin E had a much greater tumor kill from radiation therapy. 102 Radiation therapists know that the ability to kill cancer with radiation diminishes as the tumor becomes more anaerobic or hypoxic. Vitamin E seems to sensitize tumors, making them more vulnerable to radiation therapy. In cultured human cancer cells, vitamin E increased the damaging effects of radiation on tumor cells. Brain cancer cells were easier to kill once pretreated with vitamin E succinate. Tumor kill in animals receiving radiation therapy was greatly increased by pretreatment with vitamin E. Vitamin E supplements reduced the breakage of red blood cells in animals given radiation therapy. Vitamin E supplements improved the wound recovery in animals given preoperative radiation.

Vitamin E combined with vitamin K, leucovorin (anti-metabolite cancer drug), and 5FU (fluorouracil) significantly enhanced the cell growth inhibition curves for 5FU. One of the more troublesome side effects of chemotherapy is peripheral neuropathy, or a tingling numbness in the extremities. Low vitamin E status is likely to blame for peripheral neuropathy.

Oral mucositis, or sores in the mouth, is a common problem arising from the use of many chemotherapy drugs. These mouth sores are so painful that cancer patients stop eating, creating malnutrition, which really deteriorates the general health picture. Vitamin E topically applied healed 67% of cancer patients in a double-blind trial at M.D. Anderson Hospital in Houston. To use this therapy, puncture the end of a soft gelatin vitamin E capsule and spread the vitamin E oil over the mouth sore 3 times daily.

SAFETY ISSUES

Taking many times the RDA of vitamin E had some researchers worried about toxicity, so they fed 900 iu (90 times the RDA) daily to healthy college students for 12 weeks with no changes in liver, kidney, thyroid, blood clotting, or immunoglobulin levels. These results are valuable, because vitamin E inhibits the platelet aggregation that can cause stroke, heart disease, or cancer metastasis; yet it does not alter blood clotting activity. Therefore, pre-surgical patients do not need to reduce vitamin E intake for fear of not clotting during and after surgery. According to a review of the world's literature on vitamin E toxicity, there are virtually no side effects at dosages under 3,200 iu/day.

Chapter 7

Methods of Alternative Cancer Treatments

Many types of alternative treatments can be found which will be helpful for you and will be easy for you to take. Doctors may not tell you about these treatments, but you have to know about them. If you know about these kinds of treatments, it will be beneficial. Now you are going to know these kinds of treatments.

1. ***Acupuncture:*** Acupuncture is a treatment which reduces the pain of the joints. A lot of women who were suffering from joint pain and the pain were only for their breast cancer disease. Here you can get a lot of types of acupuncture method like, Xerostomia Acupuncture, Acupuncture chemotherapy, Chronic Lymphedema Acupuncture etc. You can choose anyone of these for your problem.

2. ***Gerson therapy:*** Gerson therapy is one kind of alternative therapy which was made by Max Gerson,which helps people to get a good treatment for cancer. Actually it is the therapy which only depends on the changes in nutrient intake and diet. The main features of Gerson therapy are the nutritional and biological supplements and coffee or other kinds of douche. This therapy builds up the immune system, aims at to detoxify the total body and raises the level of potassium in the cells of the body.

3. ***Yoga Therapy:*** Yoga therapy is only a practice of a person's body and not anything. This therapy helps older persons with the back pain of chronic

71

low which is very difficult to treat for all. Again it helps older persons with their muscle controlling and the joints of their body. There can be found in many types of yoga practice like, Breast cancer yoga, Aromatase Inhibitor yoga, Lung cancer yoga etc.

4. **Hypnosis:** Another complementary therapy for cancer is the hypnosis. It helps women with their breast cancer mostly. Women's take this treatment for solving their breast cancer problem. This is one of the best important therapies in the world. It has a large number of advantages for your body and to reduce the cancer from your body forever.

5. **Aromatherapy:** This therapy decreases the nausea and vomiting and anxiety which are helpful for cancer treatment. Actually the nausea and vomiting are the most symptoms of cancer for children. Symptoms can cause cancer to be difficult for the children and these symptoms can be decreased by the aromatherapy. This kind of job can be done by the acupuncture therapy also.

6. **Meditation:** Meditation means the practice of daily habit and it is also a good alternative cancer therapy. Meditation can remove the anxiety of mind which is also a treatment because the anxiety of mind can cause cancer and it is also a symptom of causing cancer.

7. **Music Therapy:** Music therapy is not a hard job at all and it can be done by only simple way. It is the job of listening to music, singing song, writing the lyrics of song etc. The music therapy can help a

person by reducing the pain and by song etc. The music therapy can help a person by reducing the pain and by controlling the nausea and vomiting.

8. **Herbal Therapy:** Again there have a therapy for alternative cancer treatment named herbal therapy which is also very important to all. It gives a real solution of cancer disease which makes a man free from cancer in its natural equipments.

9. **Light Therapy:** Again there can be found an alternative therapy named light therapy. For this therapy, different types of lights and different types of beams are needed. By using separate light beams the doctors can decrease the cancer cells easily.

10. **Magnetic Therapy:** Magnetic therapy is also one kind of alternative therapy for which different types of magnets are being used. The magnets can reduce the cancer cells and also can increase the normal programmed cells.

11. **Electrohomeopathy:** This type of therapy was invented by a person named Count Cesare Mattei. He explained that different colors of electricity can allow us to treat cancer and can kill the cancer cells. He discovered this process in the nineteenth century.

Without these types of therapies, there are plenty of therapies available in the world. You can find these treatments in your area and all over the world. So you can choose any kind of these therapies for your problem solving purpose.

Chapter 8

Successful alternative and natural therapies in the world

1. **Antineoplastic:** Antineoplastons are the peptide fractions which usually derive from the blood and urine of human body. It repairs the mis-programmed cell rather than killing these. So these are very significant not only for destroying the cancer cells but also for repairing the mis-programmed cells. So mis-programmed cells can get repaired by the antineoplastic easily and makes the body of a person free from the cancer cells. The killing of cancer cells keeps a person released from cancer.

2. **Argentinian:** This process of treatment was made by a simple mistake. When there were going on a study over breast cancer cells in a test tube. When there were going to do the test for reducing the breast cancer cells but amazingly they had got the highly decreasing of breast cancer cells which were very large than the main purpose. After that, they had started to use the technique for solving the problem of cancer.

3. **Cesium Chloride:** From the alkaline elements cesium chloride is one of the most one. It is used for increasing the pH of our body and is used as an alternate cancer. This treatment process was made by Dr. Otto Warburg and he got the Nobel Prize for cancer thrives in anaerobic showing. Cesium

chloride helps a person by killing the cancer cells and increasing the normal cells.

4. **Curcumin:** In the spice turmeric Curcumin is the active compound which also used to reduce the cancer cells. Scientists discovered curry powder which can help a person to reduce the breast cancer.

5. **Far infrared therapy:** This therapy is used to kill the cancer cells and increasing the normal well decorated cells and decreasing the side effects of conventional treatments.

6. **Germanium:** Many high concentration medicinal plants contain a versatile, health mineral which is called germanium. Actually it enhances the oxygen catalyst, electrostimulent, antioxidant and immune. Germanium is also very useful for decreasing cancer.

7. **Immune therapies:** Immunes have the capacity to fight against infections, cancer and other types of diseases. Of all age's peoples, this therapy is not open. It is only available for the middle aged persons and not for others.

8. **Fatty Acids:** The fatty acids can't be made by our body and if we want to get the fatty acids, we need to enter these into our body. Omega 3 fatty acids is the best for reducing the breast cancer. Actually we get these fatty acids from different types of foods.

9. **Oxygen Therapies:** The oxygen has also a great effect for decreasing the cancer cells from our body and for that it is called the enemy of the worst

cells. As an enemy of the worst cells it gives us relief from having cancer cells.

10. ***Psychotherapy:*** This therapy increases the belief of long living in the earth which helps cancer affected person to have self confidence. These types of therapy give a man long time living hope and also give a long time living.

Chapter 9

What are the benefits of alternative cancer therapies?

A large number of benefits can be easily found for the unconventional cancer therapies. Here you are going to know the benefits of alternative cancer therapies.

1. **Side effects:** There you will find no side effects for alternative cancer therapies and it is the most important matter for these therapies. For medical treatments, you will need to have a huge amount of medicines which may have many side effects and these effects will make you sick again. If you use in order to take the conventional therapies, the doctors may give you the prescription of having a huge amount of medicines. The huge amount of medicines has a negative effect on your health, but the alternative treatments have no effects like these.

2. **Affection:** The Affections of the alternative therapies is positive for our health and it puts its positive effect only. However, sometimes you may get some negative affects also. So it bases on your luck. But most effects of these therapies are positive. If a treatment like the conventional treatment has negative effects on your health, it will cause a lot of harm to your body. So you should choose the best service to lead the best life.

3. **Saving Money:** These kinds of therapies help a person from wasting a huge amount of money. If you take the alternate treatments, it will not take more money like the other conventional treatments. For the conventional treatments, you will need to have more money not only for the therapies but also for buying a lot of medicines. So

saving of money is totally dependent on these types of alternative therapies and gives you the best service as you wish to get.

4. **Keeping Fit:** Alternative therapies keep a person fit as like the before. These types of benefit are really important for all of us. If you want to keep yourself fit after the treatment, you can easily get the alternate treatments. The fit of the body also depends on these types of treatments. If you want to keep your body and health fit, you can take this treatment and get the real fit for your body.

5. **Spiritual Treatment:** Alternative treatments do the benefits not only for the physical conditions but also for the spiritual conditions. Therapies like yoga keep a man fit with his physical condition also. So this is also a valuable spiritual treatment also. If you want to get the heavenly peace for you, you can take the treatment easily and without having a single confusion.

These treatments will give you the best result and will bring success to kill the cancer cells from your body.

Chapter 10

Why do you need to get the alternative cancer therapies?

If you a cancer affected person and want to get a fair treatment you can easily get the treatments. The treatments have not only the great positive effects for your health but also the costs for these treatments are very low. If you are seeking for the best treatment with a minimal budget, you can take these kinds of treatments without having any kind of confusion but you have to be careful from taking a wrong treatment. Some of the natural medicines help the cancer cells to grow up instead of decreasing. So you need to be enthusiastic about these and get the best treatment with a short budget and without any confusion about the treatment. If you are seeking for the best treatment with a tiny amount of money, you need to have these types of treatments. Actually the therapies have a lot of effects to kill the cells of cancer and to increase the normal and well decorated cells. So you need to have therapies for your best purpose. Alternative treatments will bring a success for you and you will not fall for these types of problems in future. If you want to get relief from the cancer and want not to face these types of problem again, you can select the alternate therapies for your best. Only the alternate treatments can give you the best solution and for this you can choose the alternative therapies. It can give you a guarantee about solving the cancer from your body. If you take these treatments, you will get the benefit which will be distinct from the conventional treatments.

Chapter 11

Alternative Therapies Medicines

There can be found in some types of medicines for alternative cancer therapies. The medicines can be different for different types of treatments. The medicines have a lot of positive effects for cancer disease. Actually the medicines for alternative treatments are not scientifically made, but these were made by many physicians. The medicines can be herbal medicines, authentic medicines and

made by chemicals. If any medicine can be found by full of chemicals, that will not be an alternative treatment medicine. The oncologists made the medicines for the treatments of cancer only by using the natural resources. But there you will also find some medicines which are made by chemicals and without only these kinds of medicines all others are made from natural resources.

For physical therapy, and for exercise therapy, there needs some massage or some gentle techniques. These techniques are utilized to joints of therapies and deep muscles.

For acupuncture, oncologists give the instructions for medicines of the treatments. You are required to follow the instructions of the oncologists.

Again for homeopathic therapies, you will get the medicines which will be 100% pure and these will be given for your cancer cells destruction.

Again you can get some medicines for your lifestyle counseling process. Medicines can be medicine as a

80

name, but they are not the real medicine and they are the only regular practices like, physical exercises, diet, improving time of sleeping time and other types of practices.

You can get the instructions to have some minerals, vitamins and amino acids for your skin cancer and these are very accommodating for your cancer disease.

You can get some castor oil as your medicine for solving the cancer from your body and the oil has a good effect to reduce cancer.

Without these medicines, you may get a large number of medicines for your cancer. Every oncologist provides different types of medicines. So that's not a matter for you but you should be active about the medicines when you are going to get the treatments.

Chapter 12

What should you know before going to take the alternative treatments?

Many things you should know about the alternate therapies when you are going to take the therapies for your better result. If you know the matters, you will get the goal of you ultimately.

Activeness: you should be active about the oncologists who will provide you the treatments and the medicines. You should know about him/her very clearly because a lot of unqualified oncologists are also involved in these kinds of jobs.

Side effect: You should know about the side effects of the medicine which you are going to take from the oncologists because now a daze a lot of unqualified oncologists are making a lot of medicines which are made by chemicals. These kinds of medicines carry a lot of side effects to your health.

Quality of medicines: Actually many kinds of genuine medicines have some difficulties and these difficulties are very harmful for you because the medicines will increase the cancer cells instead of destroying. So you should be vigorously about these effects.

Popularity: You should know about popularity of the institution from where you are going to take the treatments. If you know that one place is very popular so you may know the cause of popularity. An institution gets popularity only by giving better service to the patients. So you should know about the popularity of the institution.

If you know about all of the things above, you will get the real benefit of the alternative cancer treatments. If you don't follow the rules, it will cause harm for you which you will know after taking the treatments. If you don't follow the rules above, your body may affect a lot of diseases. So all of the matters of the above you should know to get the best therapy.

Chapter 13

What are the differences between conventional and alternative therapies?

There can be found a lot of differences between the conventional therapies and alternative therapies. The differences are very critical but cool to find out. Here you are going to get some of the differences which you should know about must. Knowing the differences between the alternative and conventional treatments is very important for you to take the best therapy.

1. ***Definition:*** There has been a difference between the definitions of alternative and conventional cancer therapies. Conventional treatments are treatments which medicines will give by your doctor and the medicines will be 100% chemical mixed. Nevertheless, from alternative therapies many of these can be done by self and some of these needs to take help from the doctors.

2. ***Medicines:*** For the alternative therapies maximum medicines are from raw resources. On the other hand of the conventional therapies, most of the medicines are from chemicals and a scientific approach. In one speech, we can say that the alternative therapies are from natural sources and conventional therapies are of scientific methods.

3. ***Side effects:*** alternative treatments have no side effects on the human body and these are not harmful to the health of us. On the other hand,

conventional therapies have a lot of side effects for our health. So this is an essential difference between alternative therapies and conventional therapies.

4. *Science:* With conventional methods the effect of science is 100% required but for the alternative treatments the natural affects art 100% required. Without science the conventional treatments can't be done and without natural resources the alternative treatments can't be done.

5. *Money:* For conventional treatments, you will need to have a huge amount of money to get a good treatment. On the other hand, you can complete your cancer reducing therapy with a short amount of money in the alternative therapies.

There can be also some more differences found, but these differences totally depend on the persons who are going to take the treatment of reducing the cancer disease. The differences can help you differentiate between the alternative and conventional treatments. So this is really important to you to know the differences between these kinds of treatments to identify these treatments for future help.

Chapter 14

What are the disadvantages of alternative cancer treatments?

Despite the fact that the alternative treatment has a lot of benefits for us, it has some disadvantages also. Nevertheless, the disadvantages are not more than the advantages of the alternative treatments. Now you are going to show the secret weaknesses of the alternative cancer treatments.

1. **A Long Time:** The alternative treatments take a long time to give the benefits to the people's health which is not a good matter for the peoples. If a treatment takes long time to effects, that will cause harm to health. If a therapy causes some harm to our body, how can we tell these as a good one? If a treatment takes more time to give its benefit, it can't be the best one because it may harm to your health and you will get many harms instead of the benefits. So, you should be active about that matter.

2. **Growth of the cancer cell:** Sometimes many treatments medicines increase the cancer cell which is very effective for our health. The treatments increase the cancer cells instead of killing these. The growth of cancer cells can't be a good approach for a person. So this is also a bad side for this kind of treatment. For this reason you may affect some diseases and which diseases may cause you a lot of harm.

3. ***Cost:*** Although most of the medicines for alternative treatments are at a very low price but some of these price are very high. High prices medicines can take a huge amount of money from you. So you should be cautious about these types of medicines. So you should avoid these medicines to save your money and getting the best treatment.

Chapter 15

Why are a large number of people going to take the alternative treatments?

There can be found a lot of reason for attracting a huge number of people to these kinds of alternative treatments. The peoples are getting the best benefits of these kinds of therapies. By researching you can get the report that a lot of people took the conventional treatments and they have got no benefits from these kinds of treatments. After taking these kinds of treatments the people had taken the alternative treatments and they had got the actual benefit which they had wanted. Again the peoples are really satisfied with the alternative treatments regardless of the fact that these treatments are not suitable for all. The peoples can get the treatments by having a minimal amount of money and this is also a good thing for them. They can easily save their money and they can get the best treatments easily. Again the peoples who have taken the unorthodox therapies understood the real benefits of these treatments. By knowing the previous persons condition, the peoples are getting attracted by the alternative cancer therapies. The person who has taken the real benefits must have the interest to give his knowledge's on the peoples and it is also a significant reason for spreading the demand of this treatment all over the world. For all of the reason, these treatments have taken a popular place now a day.

Chapter 16

Precautions

For getting the best therapy you should take some precautionary measure. The precautionary measures will get you out of taking the harsh treatments. So these things are very important for you to know and to follow. Now you come on know about these precautionary measures.

1. ***Activeness:*** You should be active at the time of taking the treatments. If you don't pay any head to the therapies, oncologists will not pay good attention to your treatment also. So you need to have a good attention to these types of alternative cancer therapies.

2. ***Medicine:*** You should take the medicines which have no side effects on your health. If medicines contain side effects for your health, it can cause a huge amount of harm to your health. Medicines of alternative therapies often have no side effects, but if they have side effects on the medicines that will cause harm which will be more than the conventional treatments. So you should be operational about choosing the medicines of alternative therapies.

3. ***Choosing Oncologists:*** Again you should be active about choosing the oncologist with whom you are going to complete your therapy. Now a day there are a lot of unqualified oncologists can be found. Unqualified oncologists always try to give

you the bad treatments and also want to get more money from you. So you should put your best attention to this matter. Don't go to an unqualified or low experienced oncologist to take your therapies.

4. ***Dual Therapy:*** You need not to have dual therapies in a constant time because it will cause harm instead of helping you. First select the therapy and then go to the oncologists for treatments. If you take two or more than two treatments at the same time, that will cause a huge amount of harms for you. So you will feel so much of problems. To become free from all kinds of side effects, you should be active from now.

5. ***Wasting Money:*** Don't waste your money by taking a low quality therapy. You need to know the cost of the treatment first and then go for the treatments. Without knowing the real costs of the alternative treatments, you should not go forward with a single step.

6. ***Wasting time:*** Don't waste your time by having the lowest quality therapies. If you take the lowest quality therapies, it will take a long time to demonstrate its performance. For a long time treatment of the usefulness of the treatments can be going down instead of growing up your fitness. So you need to put a kind attention to this matter.

If a person knows the precautions and takes the precautionary measures, he/she will get the real benefits of having complementary treatments. The precautions can make a person enthusiastic about the treatments and can keep them fit for the future.

Chapter 17

SOME MINERALS AND CANCER

Minerals play an important role in our health and well being. We need to supplement out bodies with extra vitamins and minerals make it strong and more powerful to provide better resistance against diseases. Following are some of the essential minerals that play an important role in our fight against cancer.

Calcium - A proven protector against colon cancer, this mineral is integral for maintaining the health of bones and teeth, blood clotting, and cellular metabolism. Excellent sources include: nuts and seeds, carrot juice, dark green vegetables, salmon and sardines.

Iodine - This mineral is found in sea vegetables like kelp, dulse, and Celtic sea salt. It helps protect the body from breast cancer and is required for energy and the growth and repair of healthy tissues.

Magnesium - This mineral protects against cancer in general, maintains the pH balance of the blood, as well as aids the formation of your body's genetic material–RNA and DNA. While damaged genetic material can put you at risk for cancer, magnesium helps with the repair work. It is found in many foods, including: nuts, fish, brown rice, whole grains, and green vegetables.

Selenium - This mineral helps the body manufacture glutathione, an enzyme required for proper detoxification of the body.

Zinc - A powerful protective agent against prostate cancer, this mineral is also necessary for the formation of RNA and DNA and a healthy immune system.

Chapter 18

VITAMIN B17 – THE UNTOLD STORY

Although, not new to the world of cancer treatment, thousands of people around the globe have used, and are still using a key active ingredient found in apricot pits and known as Amygdalin. Laetrile is the man-made or synthetic version of Amygdalin; it is also known as Vitamin B17. There is a tiny amount of organic cyanide present in this vitamin, and therefore it shows promising results in fighting against cancer.

Vitamin B17 remains a mystery till to date, despite so much research is carried out on the effectiveness of this vitamin to effectively destroy cancer cells in earlier stages of the disease.

Mode of Action

The laetrile molecules when come in contact with the caner cells are broken down into two molecules; one molecule of hydrogen cyanide and one of benzaldehyde. Earlier it was believed that it is the hydrogen cyanide molecule that takes an active part in destroying the cancer cells, however latest research reveals that it is actually the benzaldehyde molecule that does the work.

Although the use of Amygdalin is not new to the world we live in, ancient Egyptians have used bitter almonds for treating various diseases. Some historical finding recovered from various Egyptian ruins mention the use of "aqua amigdalorum" for successfully treating some skin tumors.

A well-systematic and well-documented study about the role of Vitamin B17 in curing cancer did not start till the first half of the past century. Scientists were able to extract a white crystalline substance from the almond oil and they called it AMYGDALIN (meaning almond). Ever since the discovery and extraction of this cancer-fighting agent from the almond and apricot seeds, there has been great controversy behind the effectiveness of Amygdalin in treating cancer. Even though a number of people have enjoyed great success in treating their cancer with this active ingredient, some governmental agencies like FDA as well as other major drug manufactures have discredited amygdalin (Vitamin B17).

The cultural evidence

Eskimos, Hunzas and Abkasians have a long history of using food items that are rich in Vitamin B17. A close examination of their life reveals that there are very rare incidences of caner reported in their population. Is it just a coincidence or evidence about the effectiveness of Vitamin B17 in preventing the occurrence of cancer in our body?

List of foods rich in Vitamin B17

If Eskimos and Hunzas can defeat cancer by eating diet rich in Vitamin B17, there is no reason you can do the same, however you need to know what kind of food items contain huge amounts of this vitamin. Following is a list of foods that can offer you plenty of this cancer fighting and cancer preventing vitamin:

Fruit Kernels or seeds - there are certain fruit kernels or seeds which contain the highest amounts of Vitamin B17; these include apricot, peach, almond, apple, plum, cherry, pear and prune.

Berries - vitamin B17 is present in some amount in almost all of the wild berries, such as cranberry, blackberry, raspberry, chokeberry and strawberry

Grasses - certain grasses such as wheat grass, aquatic, milkweed, alfalfa, white Dover, acacia and Sudan contain this vitamin

Beans - such as chickpeas, scarlet runner, Burma, lima, and mung also contain plenty of vitamin B17

Nuts - nuts, such as almond, walnuts, cashew, and macadamia are another good source of this vitamin.

Seeds - certain seeds such as sesame, Chia and flax can also offer plenty of Vitamin B17.

Grains - you can also supply your body with this Vitamin by including certain grains, such as brown rice, millet, oats, rye, barley and flax in your daily diet.

Some other forms of Vitamin B17

In the section above, a list of food items were shared with you that provide the body the much needed Vitamin B17 (laetrile), however besides these natural sources, you can also take laetrile in the following forms:

- ✓ As laetrile tablets
- ✓ As laetrile injections
- ✓ As a liquid that is injected through the rectum
- ✓ As a skin lotion

Before taking laetrile in any of the above mentioned forms, it is necessary that you consult an expert. There is certain amount (dosage) of laetrile that you can take or inject in your body. Excessive dosage of this vitamin in the body may increase the levels of cyanides, which can be a risky situation.

If you are considering taking laetrile tablets or injections, you also need to supplement your body by taking high doses of other vitamins and also eat a healthy diet to enjoy better recovery.

Some Side effects

Although it is a completely natural ingredient and does not harm the body in any way or form, however over dosage of this vitamin can result in the increased levels of cyanide in the body, and as a result you may experience certain side effects. Some of the typical side effects associated with taking excessive laetrile are:

- ✓ Low blood pressure
- ✓ Headaches
- ✓ Liver damage
- ✓ Fever
- ✓ Dropping eyelids
- ✓ Dizziness
- ✓ Damage to nerve endings
- ✓ Loss of balance
- ✓ Coma
- ✓ Death

Precaution

The presence of cyanide make laetrile application very tricky, you need to monitor your dosage to keep cyanides levels in the body at certain levels, over dosage may lead to coma and/or even death. It is estimated that eating 50-60 apricot kernels or taking more than 50g or laetrile in the form of injections or tablets can lead to death. If you have chosen to go with the laetrile tablets or injections, you need to stay away from eating foods rich in amygdalin.

Keeping in constant contact with your doctor is therefore very important, whether you prefer the conventional treatment option of alternative treatment. You should share the outcomes of your treatments with your doctor frequently and in case you observe any serious side reaction, you need to bring those into his/her notice and seek medical assistance without any delays.

Chapter 19

Following Your Intuition

In many ways, humans have lost touch with their instincts. We used to be hunters and gatherers—people who could sense when a storm was coming or feel when a grizzly bear was nearby. Our sense of smell also used to be much more highly developed, as it expertly guided us toward safe food and away from poisons. When we got sick, we listened to our bodies by allowing a fever to burn off the illness and by not eating for a few days. Today, things are quite different. We rely on whatever The Weather Channel tells us, we eat whatever processed foods we find in the supermarket, and we take whatever medicine our doctors give us.

There are two potential problems with relying on such outside sources of information, though. First, the sources could be wrong. For example, commercials in the 1950s showed doctors in white coats promoting the health benefits of cigarettes, while margarine—with all its trans fat—was touted as a "healthier" alternative to butter. These examples show us that others do not always know what is best for us. Second, instincts are a lot like multiplication tables: if you don't use them, you lose them. Along this line, researchers believe that our sense of smell has diminished over the past few centuries because we no longer need it to survive, as safe food is now so abundant in our grocery stores and restaurants. However, by not keeping our sense of smell well honed, we have lost the ability to detect new toxins in our environment, such as cancer-causing chemicals in our food, air, and water.

And then there is intuition, that famous sixth sense or instinct that seems to come from a deeper place. Many people would argue that we have lost this as well. For example, there are records of our ancestors following the intuitive guidance they received from dreams, and thousand-year-old yogic texts describing meditation exercises that can help increase our intuitive abilities. Although I was not expecting it, "following your intuition" has ended up being one of the nine most common factors of Radical Remission among the people I research. I remember, on my fiftieth or so interview of these survivors, thinking, There it is again! However, now that I have done further research on intuition, I am no longer surprised but thrilled to have been reintroduced to this "lost" sense of ours, which has the ability to help steer us away from danger and onto the path of recovery.

In this chapter, we will first explore three aspects of intuition as described by the Radical Remission survivors I study, followed by the story of a woman whose intuition played a key role in the healing of her pancreatic cancer. Finally, you will find a list of simple action steps that you can start taking right now to help you rediscover your innate, sixth sense of intuition.

The Body Knows What It Needs To Heal

The Radical Remission survivors I study believe the body has an innate, intuitive knowledge about what it needs in order to heal, and it can often also let you know why it got sick in the first place. It is because of this that many Radical Remission survivors believe it is vital to check in with your intuition before making any sort of healing plan. Interestingly, this belief goes against typical Western medicine thinking, which usually removes patients from the planning process while the expert doctors determine what is wrong with their bodies and how to fix it.

One of the alternative healers I studied, who firmly believes the body intuitively knows what it needs in order to heal, is "Maya" Karen Sorensen, a BodyTalk practitioner from Hawaii. BodyTalk is a form of energy medicine that uses the principles of energy kinesiology and muscle monitoring to figure out where the root problems are located in the body, what's causing them, and how they can be released quickly. In this way, Maya works directly with the intuition of her patients' bodies. She describes her healing in this way:

BodyTalk is speed healing, because the body wants to be whole and knows how to be whole. But sometimes it needs to be reconnected to its innate knowledge. The body can heal very instantly; it's our belief system that makes us think that it takes a long time to heal. Using energy medicine kind of bypasses the belief system, because it taps into the client's deeper, innate wisdom of the body.

Similarly, another healer I researched believes the body naturally knows how to return to wellness. Derek O'Neill is a Radical Remission cancer survivor himself who later became a healer and now encourages the cancer patients with whom he works to access their intuition:

If the mind is allowed to quiet down, it will know what it needs to do in order to get well again. It's a built-in system that every being has. . . . So, cancer is actually only a messenger. It's not a be-all and end-all, in my opinion. It's a messenger to say that something has gone negative, something is out of alignment. Find out what that something is, and you will note that the energetics of your own body will begin to correct that system.

Once cancer patients become aware of the ways in which their lives have become out of balance, Derek encourages them to make addressing those imbalances an integral part of their healing plan.

The Many Ways To Access Intuition

The second aspect of following intuition is that there is no one "right" way to access your intuition. For some people, their intuition comes to them through an internal voice of deep knowing; for others, it comes more as a physical feeling in their bodies, such as a warning pang in their guts; for still others, their intuition speaks to them in their dreams, their meditations, their journals, or through serendipitous "coincidences," such as bumping into a friend who told them exactly the information they needed to hear at exactly the right time. All these methods are valid ways to access your intuition, and the more often you access it, the clearer the messages will be.

One Radical Remission survivor who used dreams to access her intuition for healing was Wanda Easter Burch. When Wanda was forty-two, she began having vivid dreams warning her that she had breast cancer, even though her mammogram was clear and an ultrasound was inconclusive. Nevertheless, she insisted on having a needle biopsy, and that is when her dreams proved to be true: she indeed had aggressive breast cancer.

After her diagnosis, Wanda began to study dream interpretation more deeply, and she blended meditation, drawing, and poetry into her conventional treatments of surgery and chemotherapy. She describes her use of intuitive dream work this way:

Before and after my radical surgery and aggressive chemotherapy, my dreams presented images that provided personal, creative material. Dreaming—and selective mining of dream imagery—empowers the mind, spirit, and body. Dream work encourages dialogue with the inner physician—a constantly streaming, two-way message center that speaks to us, knows us best, and offers gateways to healing beyond the hospital or doctor's office. There are no artificial boundaries in a dream, nor a limit on the varieties of creative and healing artistic expression that can emerge.

Wanda used dreams to help her figure out which foods to eat during chemotherapy, which emotional patterns to release, and which conventional medicine treatments to consider. She has now been cancer-free for over twenty-three years.

Another Radical Remission survivor who used dreams to access her intuition was Nancy. On May 1, 2006, Nancy was just about to turn sixty-five when biopsy results came back showing that she had breast cancer. Her tumor was too big for a lumpectomy, so her doctor recommended a full mastectomy followed by radiation therapy and the estrogen-reducing pill tamoxifen. However, Nancy's intuition told her to try alternative methods first, so she politely turned down the surgery and all other conventional treatments. Listening to her intuition, especially her dreams, turned out to be a pivotal part of her healing:

On May 5 [four days after her diagnosis] I had two dreams. . . . In the second dream, my son-in-law was looking for Spray 'n Wash to treat a dark red stain on our old, well-worn tablecloth. I told him where it was, but he couldn't find it. After much searching, I found it right on the table and went ahead and sprayed the stains, which began to dissolve. In real life, [he] is a skilled orthopedic surgeon. I believe my intuition was telling me that I could heal this cancer without surgery, but it would take time and effort, and I'd find the solution right there in my own, well-worn, much-used, much-loved body.

After putting together a healing plan that encompassed dietary, exercise, herbal, emotional, spiritual, and energetic treatments, Nancy was declared cancer-free by her doctor just sixteen months later. She remains cancer-free to this day and is certainly glad she listened to her intuition.

Everyone Has A Different Change They Need To Make

The third aspect of following intuition is the idea that every person may have a different change they need to make in order to heal his or her cancer, and that is why checking in with your intuition can be so vital to your recovery. For example, I met one cancer survivor whose intuition told her she had to quit the job she hated in order to get well. Another person's intuition told him he had to move to a different climate in order to heal, and yet another person's intuition told her she needed to start exercising again. The alternative healers whose work I study agree with this idea of trusting your own unique intuition. They tell me repeatedly that every person has a different change they must make in order to restore balance to their systems. For some people, that may mean changing their diets, but for others, it may mean changing their marriages.

This idea goes against current Western medicine thinking, which aims to find a single cause for a disease and a single cure for it. In the case of bacterial infections, this goal is realistic: we can try to determine the single bacterium that has infected the body and then try to develop a single antibiotic that will destroy that bacterium. However, with a more complex disease such as cancer, which has already been shown to have multiple causes (toxins, viruses, bacteria, genetic mutation, mitochondria damage, etc.), finding a single cure may not be so realistic. In this case, then, it would make sense that some cancer patients would benefit greatly from making a particular change (e.g., radical diet change) while other cancer patients would not.

That's when intuition can be extremely helpful: when you are trying to figure out the particular change your body-mind-spirit needs in order to heal. Gemma Bond is a Radical Remission survivor who was diagnosed with ovarian cancer in 2011. After agreeing to a hysterectomy, during which her uterus and ovaries were surgically removed, her intuition strongly told her to refuse the recommended chemotherapy. Instead, she began exploring alternative therapies, such as intravenous vitamin C and ozone therapy. She also read as many books as she could find about alternative cancer treatment:

In one of the many books I have read, the author—a cancer survivor himself—suggests that anybody with cancer sit quietly with their cancer and then ask why it has come, and then ask it what needs to be done in order for it to leave. So, I did that. I sat quietly with my cancer and I thought, Why have you come? I had led such a healthy physical life - I'd exercised, I'd eaten organic, I'd fed my four children what I thought was great, healthy food . . . but the answer really screamed back at me, You have no joy in your life! You always have this really big to-do list, but where is your joy? I had looked after my physical health, but I had really neglected my emotional health. And so, that has become the thing that I have worked on most in my healing, my emotional health rather than my physical health—although I have tweaked that as well.

Thanks to this intuitive insight, Gemma began addressing her emotional health by adding more joy to her life and deepening her connection with spirit. Only six months after her diagnosis, her tumor markers were back down to within a normal range, and she is still cancer-free to this day.

An energy healer based in London's Hale Clinic named Danira Caleta purposefully begins teaching cancer patients how to access their intuition in her very first healing session with them, so they can understand the specific ways in which their health has gone out of balance:

I teach [my patients] to actually turn on that switch in the unconscious, which is faith. In quantum healing, they call it "the doctor within." It's like a light switch. And I teach them how to do this. . . . Your body's on your side. It does actually give you a warning. It does tell us, "Look, there's something not quite right here." But most people don't listen and they put it off, thinking, Oh, it'll just go away. So, one has to listen to one's body. . . . Cancer is about a journey to teach us many things about ourselves. It really forces us to examine how we're living.

In Danira's opinion, when you use your intuition to listen to your body to figure out the particular change you need to make, healing will follow naturally.

The Research On Intuition

While unfortunately there has not been a lot of research conducted on intuition specifically, researchers have made important discoveries that relate indirectly to intuition. The first discovery was that humans appear to have two very different "operating systems." System one is the quick, instinctual, and often subconscious way of operating; it is controlled by the right side of the brain and by other parts of the brain that have been around since prehistoric times, known as the "limbic" and "reptilian" parts. System two is the slower, more analytical, and conscious way of operating; it is controlled by the left side of the brain and by newer parts of the brain that have only developed since prehistoric times, also known as the "neocortex." Researchers have found that intuition is part of system one, which is why it comes on so rapidly and often does not make rational sense to us. In other words, intuitive decisions are not things we think through carefully, with reason, but rather choices that arise quickly, out of instinct.

Second, scientists have discovered that over a hundred million neurons— the type of cells found in your brain— also exist inside the human digestive tract, which explains why people often say they have a "gut feeling" about something. This is because the gut, with all its millions of neurons, can actually think and feel just like the brain can. Even more interesting has been the discovery that this "second brain" in your gut can act independently of the brain, meaning that your gut can decide to stop digesting food and send you a sudden, intuitive pang of warning without any input from your brain. So far, the gut is the only organ that has been discovered to have this independent operating ability.

All of this leads us to the fact that we now have a scientific explanation for why people so often decide to go with their gut when making a decision. People also feel pangs of anxiety or stress in their guts, but this is also related to intuition, because it is the body's way of saying,

"Stop what you're doing. This situation is not healthy for you." So, your gut can communicate that it wants you to remove yourself from a stressful or anxious situation, just as it can communicate to you that that one is the house you should buy.

But why, exactly, should we trust a gut instinct? One reason is because researchers have found that system one often knows the right answer long before system two does. For example, in one study, researchers asked their subjects to play a card game where the goal was to win the most money. What the study subjects did not realize, however, is that the game was rigged from the start. There were two stacks of cards to choose from; one was rigged to provide big wins followed by big losses, while the other deck was set up to provide small gains but almost no losses. It took about fifty cards before the subjects said they had a hunch about which deck was safer and about eighty cards before they could actually explain the difference between the two decks. What is most fascinating is that after only ten cards, the sweat glands on the subjects' palms opened slightly every time they reached for a card in the dangerous deck. It was also around the tenth card that the subjects started to favor the safer deck, without being consciously aware they were doing so. 6 In other words, long before the analytical brain could explain what was going on, the subjects' bodily intuition knew where there was danger and guided them toward safety.

A similar study looked at people's ability to predict whether a picture was behind curtain number one or curtain number two (though this was done on a computer, so there were no actual curtains involved). Just like with the card study, the researchers measured the subjects' subtle physiological responses. Remarkably, they found that the subjects' bodies were able to predict the correct curtain two to three seconds before the computer had even decided which curtain to use. The subjects did not always follow through with what their slightly sweaty palms were telling them to do, but the slightly sweaty palms were almost always right; in fact, they even had the ability to predict the future (by those two to three seconds). For gamblers who would like to have the ability to predict a certain card, this study suggests they should work on heightening their sense of intuition to such a degree that they can recognize when the sweat glands on their palms have opened up.

Finally, there is another set of studies that gives us yet another reason we should trust our intuition. These studies have found that, when it comes to making major life decisions, such as which house to buy or which person to marry, trusting your intuition leads to better outcomes than trusting your logical, thinking brain. In one such study, car buyers who had plenty of time to pore over all the information about their various car choices were later found to be satisfied with their purchase only 25 percent of the time. Meanwhile, those buyers who made a quick, intuitive decision about their car purchases were found to be satisfied with their purchases 60 percent of the time. In three similar experiments, subjects were either given time to think about a complex problem or distracted and then asked to make a quick decision. Across the board, the subjects who were asked to make quick, intuitive decisions were the ones who made the best decisions overall. In other words, these studies indicate that it is best to trust your intuition when it comes to making complex life decisions, while it is better to use your slower, more analytical brain for solving simpler problems.

While I was surprised to have intuition come up over and over again during my research of Radical Remission cancer survivors, these studies tell me that I should not be surprised at all, because our intuition often knows what's best for us even when our thinking minds do not yet understand what's going on. That's because intuition operates from the part of our brains that developed at a time when hidden dangers could jump out at us at any moment, such as a tiger hiding behind bushes. This part of the brain became highly skilled at sensing immediate danger as well as places of safety. However, because most of us now (thankfully) live a relatively safe day-to- day existence, that part of our brains is not triggered very often, and when it is, we are not familiar with it, so we tend to ignore its messages. However, we all still have it, and the Radical Remission survivors I study have learned how to harness its power.

IN TODAY'S WORLD, talking about following your intuition can make people think you are "woo-woo." That is certainly what happened with Susan Koehler. Susan's intuition came roaring up inside her when she was diagnosed with stage 4 pancreatic cancer, and everyone thought she was crazy for listening to it. As you read her complete healing story, I invite you to think about times in your life when your intuition has suddenly kicked in. Have you ever felt a pang in your stomach that made you pick up the phone and call someone just at the right time? Did the next major step in your life ever come to you in a flash of inspired creativity or through a beautiful dream? As you will see in Susan's story, we shouldn't ignore these flashes of intuition, because they often have important -perhaps even life-saving - information to tell us.

Conclusion

According to the latest research published in the Journal of Patient Safety, as much as 400,000 patients die every year in US hospitals alone, due to lack of research, or medical negligence. Now compare it with the Vietnam War which lasted for about 10 years and contributed to the death of about 1,100,000 people all together, that comes out to be 110,000 per year deaths, which is still much lower as compared to the deaths caused by the medical profession.

Anyone who is thinking about chemo or radiation therapy which offers only 4% success rates, need to read this book to find out the remaining 96% options.

It is quite understandable that people who are faced with this terrible disease are ready to go to any length and try any option that offers them some kind of hope for life. However, it is also equally important to do your home work thoroughly before you decide which treatment option is the best for you.

Consultations with your doctors, your close friends, your family members and most importantly with cancer victors need to be given prime importance. Once you are done with all the consultations, you can easily make up your mind whether to go for the conventional, complementary or alternative approach.

Religion also plays an important role in our lives, and can provide us the answers to the most of the unsolved mysteries of life. A clue about cancer treatment and cancer prevention as evident in the religious books is quoted as under:

Reference: Genesis 1:29

Then God said, "I give you every seed-bearing plant on the face of the whole earth and every tree that has fruit with seed in it. They will be yours for food."

Certain other food items are also referred in Quran, which are quoted to provide healing and cure to any kind of disease on earth, except death. These food items include fig, olive oil, dates, and pomegranate.

An ending note, no one has witnessed or read a verified case of someone dying of eating apricot seeds. There is so much information available out there, in the end it is you who has to decide which option is more close to the nature, safest and offer better long term benefits to you and your body.

www.ingramcontent.com/pod-product-compliance
Lightning Source LLC
Chambersburg PA
CBHW021439210526
45463CB00002B/577